组织胚胎实验学
（第二版）

陈永珍　黄晓燕　林巍巍　主编

科学出版社

北京

内 容 简 介

本书为中英文双语组织学与胚胎学实验教材,共有 23 章实验内容,其中组织学 18 章,胚胎学 5 章。在每章开头设有"学习要点",每章(除第一章外)末尾设有"复习思考题""图片思考题",便于学生掌握重点、自学和复习。在实验内容中对每张组织切片的学习都提出要求识别的知识点,培养学生实际观察切片的能力。此外,本书书末附有组织学与胚胎学专业词汇中英文对照,以帮助学生学习和掌握专业英文词汇。另在书末附有 146 幅彩色图片,其中组织学部分采用光镜下组织切片的彩色图片,并附有英文描述和标注;胚胎学部分以国内常用的胚胎各期模型为主。本书组织学部分在第一版基础上增加了主要观察的切片,以二维码形式体现,用于观察组织学全景数字切片扫描显微图像。

本书适合普通高等医药院校医学类各专业使用,也适用于留学生医学教育。

图书在版编目(CIP)数据

组织胚胎实验学 / 陈永珍,黄晓燕,林巍巍主编.
—2 版. —北京:科学出版社,2019.5(2023.1重印)
ISBN 978 – 7 – 03 – 061006 – 5

Ⅰ.①组… Ⅱ.①陈…②黄…③林… Ⅲ.①人体组织学-人体胚胎学-实验 Ⅳ.①R329.1 – 33

中国版本图书馆 CIP 数据核字(2019)第 067399 号

责任编辑:闵 捷 / 责任校对:谭宏宇
责任印制:黄晓鸣 / 封面设计:殷 靓

科学出版社 出版

北京东黄城根北街 16 号
邮政编码:100717
http://www.sciencep.com

南京展望文化发展有限公司排版

苏州市古得堡数码印刷有限公司印刷
科学出版社发行 各地新华书店经销

*

2014 年 7 月第 一 版 开本:787×1092 1/16
2019 年 5 月第 二 版 印张:10 插页:14
2023 年 1 月第九次印刷 字数:234 000

定价:40.00 元
(如有印装质量问题,我社负责调换)

《组织胚胎实验学》(第二版)
编委会

主 编

陈永珍　黄晓燕　林巍巍

副主编

余水长　李冬梅　郑　英
黄少萍　孙　申　陈　雪

编　委

（按姓氏笔画排序）

丁卫东 （南京大学）	王　晖 （南京医科大学）
王　蕾 （徐州医科大学）	孙　申 （徐州医科大学）
李　芳 （苏州大学）	李　奕 （南通大学）
李　颖 （苏州大学）	李冬梅 （南京大学）
吴　坚 （南通大学）	余水长 （苏州大学）
张于娟 （苏州大学）	陈　雪 （江南大学）
陈永珍 （苏州大学）	林巍巍 （南通大学）
岳海源 （扬州大学）	郑　英 （扬州大学）
姚　健 （南通大学）	郭　辉 （江南大学）
黄少萍 （东南大学）	黄晓燕 （南京医科大学）
韩晓冬 （南京大学）	程建青 （江南大学）
傅　奕 （苏州大学）	魏剑锋 （徐州医科大学）

第二版前言

《组织胚胎实验学》(第二版)是在第一版教材使用近 5 年后,听取江苏省八所医学院校意见的基础上进行的再版。再版的宗旨是使本教材适应我国当前实施的临床医学实验教学改革、卓越医师培养计划和医学留学生教学的需要。使教材尽量体现出科学性、先进性和启发性的教学模式,致力于医学生理论联系实践、临床思维和能力的培养,达到早临床、多临床和反复临床的目的。

本教材第一版以简单扼要、实用性强和便于自学等特点受到广大师生的欢迎,第二版保持前一版的特色,并在编写内容和质量上有所改进和提高。

(1)增加组织学全景数字切片扫描显微图像。将组织学各个章节主要观察的切片,采用二维码的形式,建立了"全景数字切片扫描显微图像资源库"。学生通过扫描相应切片附带的二维码,即可直接进入此资源库相应的全景数字切片扫描显微图像,并能在手机上观察更多、更大视野的图像,使手机具有"便携式显微镜"的功能。

(2)在组织学与胚胎学各个章节增加图片复习题,建立了"组织学与胚胎学图片复习题资源库",学生通过扫描每章后的二维码,即可进入此资源库,方便学生进行相应章节主要知识点的练习和巩固。

(3)根据在第一版教材使用过程中征求得到的各方面意见和建议,进行了中英文和图片的修正。

《组织胚胎实验学》再版过程中,各参编学校同行专家和老师付出了大量的心血,并得到了上海梦之路数字科技有限公司、苏州大学医学部和苏州大学医学部基础医学与生物科学学院的大力支持,苏州大学医学部人体解剖与组织胚胎学系余水长老师在"全景数字切片扫描显微图像资源库"和"组织学与胚胎学图片复习题资源库"建设过程中,付出了艰辛的工作,在此一并表示衷心的感谢!

由于我们专业水平有限,经验不足,如有错误和不妥之处,恳请同行专家、广大师生及其他读者批评指正,以便我们进一步提高教材质量,使其更加符合教学规律和人才培养的需要。

《组织胚胎实验学》(第二版)编委会

2019 年 1 月

第一版前言

　　《组织胚胎实验学》是在江苏省七所医学院校的齐心协力下完成的。宗旨是使本教材适应我国当前实施的临床医学实验教学改革、卓越医师培养计划和医学留学生教学的需要。通过实验教学引导学生主动学习；提高学生观察、分析问题、解决问题和创新的能力；培养学生科学的思维方法和严谨的科学作风，更好地满足高等学校培养适应 21 世纪需要的高质量人才的需求。

　　本教材有以下几个特点：

　　（1）本教材为双语版，全书共有 23 章内容，其中组织学 18 章，胚胎学 5 章。每章中文版和英文版相间排列，方便国内外学生阅读理解。

　　（2）本教材每个章节设有学习要点和复习思考题，使学生对每个章节的主要内容一目了然，便于学生学习时掌握重点；每张组织切片的实验内容中增加要求识别的知识点，便于学生课前预习和课后复习。

　　（3）本教材附录一有组织胚胎学专业词汇中英文对照，方便学生专业英语的学习。

　　（4）本教材附录二的组织胚胎学彩色图谱为全英文说明图解，附有胚胎学的图片，彩色图谱中共有 146 张图片，引导学生观看组织切片。

　　（5）本教材可作为普通高等医学院校的双语教材，适合高等医药院校七年制、五年制和留学生使用。根据教学计划学时数的多少以及不同专业的具体要求，可对实验内容进行合理取舍。

　　本教材使用原教材的中英文对照词汇及彩色图谱，在此谨向原主编徐昌芬教授及其他主编和所有编委表示深切的敬意和感谢！在编写过程中得到各参编学校同行专家和老师的帮助和支持，在此表示衷心的感谢！

　　由于专业水平有限，经验不足，本书难免有错误和不妥之处，恳请同行专家、广大师生及其他读者批评指正，以便进一步提高本教材的质量。

《组织胚胎实验学》编委会

2014 年 2 月

目　录

第一章

绪　论

学习要点

☞ 了解研究组织学与胚胎学的常用技术。
☞ 了解石蜡切片的一般制作方法。
☞ 掌握 HE 染色步骤,嗜酸性、嗜碱性的含义。
☞ 了解光镜和电镜下常用的长度单位。

实 验 内 容

(一) 石蜡切片的一般制作方法

1. 取材
(1) 可取自人的活检、手术切除所获组织,也可取自动物组织。取材后应尽早固定。
(2) 组织块大小一般为 $1.0 \text{ cm} \times 1.0 \text{ cm} \times 0.3 \text{ cm}$,若组织块太厚,则影响固定。

2. 固定
(1) 目的:防止组织自溶及细菌性腐败,并使柔软组织适当硬化。
(2) 组织取出后,立即入固定液,常用固定液为乙醇或甲醛。所用固定液的量应为所取组织体积的 5～10 倍,足以完全覆盖所取组织。
(3) 固定时间:依组织块大小、固定液性质而定,一般为室温 12～24 h。

3. 水洗
(1) 目的:清除残留固定液,以免影响染色。
(2) 流水冲洗,一般为 12～24 h。

4. 脱水
(1) 目的:将组织中水分除去,以便透明剂和石蜡渗入。
(2) 常用脱水剂:乙醇,浓度逐渐提高,以避免组织块急剧收缩。
(3) 脱水顺序:50%→60%→70%→80%→90%→95%→无水乙醇①→无水乙醇②在每级乙醇中停留时间为 6～12 h。

5. 透明
(1) 目的:透明剂置换乙醇,以便包埋时石蜡易于浸入组织。
(2) 常用透明剂:二甲苯。
(3) 先将组织块置于无水乙醇与二甲苯(1∶1)混合液中浸泡 0.5～2 h,然后将组织块移至二甲苯中再浸泡 0.5～1 h。

6.包埋

(1) 目的:提高组织块硬度。

(2) 常用包埋剂:石蜡。

(3) 将组织块置于熔化石蜡(58～60℃)中,渗透 1～1.5 h,然后再置于包埋框中,待冷却。

7.切片

(1) 将含有组织块的蜡块用切片机上的刀制作切片。

(2) 切片厚度一般为 4～6 μm。

8.染色

(1) 目的:使本来无色的各种组织成分染上不同颜色而便于观察。

(2) 染色剂多种多样,常用染色剂为苏木素和伊红,该染色法称 HE 染色(详见 HE 染色步骤)。

9.封固

(1) 目的:使切片能较长期保存。

(2) 常用封固剂:中性树胶。

(3) 在染色的切片上滴加一滴树胶,盖上盖玻片。

(二) HE 染色步骤

(1) 切片浸入二甲苯 10 min,借以溶去石蜡。

(2) 经 100% →90%→ 80% → 70%梯度乙醇各 5～10 min 去除二甲苯。

(3) 蒸馏水 5 min 去除乙醇。

(4) 置于苏木素(碱性染料)染液中数分钟。

(5) 流水冲洗,置入温水直至切片变蓝。

(6) 置于 95%乙醇中 10 min。

(7) 置于伊红(酸性染料)染液中约 20 s。

(8) 置于 95%乙醇中 10 min。

(9) 置于 100%乙醇中 2 次,各 10 min。

(10) 待切片干燥后封固。

(傅　奕　李　颖)

Chapter 1

INTRODUCTION

Learning Points

☞ To understand the common techniques used in the study of histology and embryology.
☞ To understand the general methods of making paraffin section.
☞ To grasp the steps of HE staining and the concept of eosinophilia and basophilia.
☞ To understand the units of measurement applied in light and electron microscopy.

Part I   Experiment Contents

1. General methods of making paraffin section

A. Material drawing

(1) Tissues, obtained from human biopsy and a surgical operation, or from animal's tissue should be collected freshly and fixed immediately.

(2) The size of the tissue block is generally 1.0 cm× 1.0 cm × 0.3 cm, because the fixation will be affected if the tissue blocks are too thick and too large.

B. Fixation

(1) The purpose of fixation is to prevent tissue digestion by enzymes (autolysis) or bacteria and make the soft tissue harden properly.

(2) Put the tissue block into the fixative reagent immediately after drawing. The most common fixative is ethanol or formaldehyde. The volume of fixative should be 5 to 10 times of tissue block, to make sure the tissue block can be submerged completely.

(3) The fixing time is determined by the size of the tissue block and the nature of the fixative, and is generally for 12 to 24 hours in room temperature.

C. Washing

(1) The purpose of washing is to remove the residual fixative reagent so as not to affect the staining.

(2) Wash in running water, usually for 12 to 24 hours.

D. Dehydration

(1) The purpose of dehydration is to strip away the remaining water, and facilitate the infiltration of clearing agents and paraffin into the tissue.

(2) Ethanol is commonly used as dehydration reagent. The concentration of ethanol is gradually increased to avoid sharp contraction of the tissue block.

(3) The processes of dehydration are as follows: 50% → 60% → 70% → 80% → 90% → 95% → unhydrous ethanol ① → unhydrous ethanol ②, 6 to 12 hours for each step.

E. Clearing

(1) The purpose of the clearing is to increase the light transmittance of the tissue, by replacing the dehydrator with clearing agent in the tissue making it easy for paraffin to infiltrate into the tissue.

(2) The xylene is commonly used as clearing agent.

(3) Firstly, to immerse the tissue in the mixture of absolute ethanol and xylene (1 : 1) for 0.5 to 2 hours, and then in xylene for 0.5 to 1 hours.

F. Embedding

(1) The purpose of embedding is to improve the hardness of the tissue.

(2) The paraffin is commonly used as embedding medium.

(3) Firstly, to immerse the tissue in the melted paraffin (58 to 60℃) for 1 to 1.5 hours, and then place it into a mould, waiting for cooling.

G. Sectioning

(1) The block of paraffin containing the tissue is sectioned by the steel blade of the microtome.

(2) The slice is generally for 4 to 6 μm thick.

H. Staining

(1) The purpose of staining is to observe the tissue easily by coloring the various components of the tissue differently which are colorless originally.

(2) There are a variety of staining reagents, among which the hematoxylin and eosin are commonly used and such staining method is called HE staining (see "Steps of HE Staining").

I. Mounting

(1) The purpose of mounting is for long-term preservation.

(2) Neutral balsam is commonly used for mounting.

(3) Basically, a drop of neutral balsam is placed on the section and then the coverslip is placed on it.

2. Steps of HE Staining

(1) The slides are placed in xylene for 10 minutes to dissolve the paraffin.

(2) To remove the remaining xylene by graded ethanol, 100%, 90%, 80% and 70%, 5 to 10 minutes for each.

(3) To rinse the slides in distilled water for 5 minutes.

(4) To immerse the slides in the hematoxylin (a basic dye) for a few minutes.

(5) To wash the slides in running water and then put it into warm water till the color of the tissues turns blue.

(6) To rinse the slides in 95% ethanol for 10 minutes.

(7) To immerse the slides in eosin (an acidic dye) for about 20 seconds.

(8) To rinse the slides in 95% ethanol again for 10 minutes.

(9) To rinse the slides in 100% ethanol twice, 10 minutes for each step.

(10) To mount the slides after drying.

(Fu Yi, Li Ying)

第二章

上 皮 组 织

学习要点

- ☞ 上皮组织的一般特点和分类。
- ☞ 各种被覆上皮的结构特点和功能。
- ☞ 上皮细胞各面的特殊结构和功能。
- ☞ 腺上皮和腺的概念。
- ☞ 外分泌腺和内分泌腺的概念。

一、实 验 内 容

单层扁
平上皮

（一）单层扁平上皮

1. 染色　　HE。

（1）低倍镜：

1）观察部位在脾表面。

2）可见脾表面一层排列整齐的扁平细胞,核呈紫蓝色,即单层扁平上皮。

（2）高倍镜：

1）细胞扁薄。

2）胞质极少,含核的部分略厚。

3）细胞核扁平,长轴与脾表面平行。

2. 要求识别

（1）上皮细胞的形状和排列。

（2）细胞核。

（3）细胞质。

单层立
方上皮

（二）单层立方上皮

1. 染色　　HE。

（1）低倍镜：

1）观察部位在肾髓质的肾小管。

2）可见大量肾小管断面,腔壁衬以单层立方上皮。

（2）高倍镜：

1）细胞立方形。

2）胞质淡红色。

3）胞核圆形，位于细胞中央。

2．要求识别

（1）上皮细胞的形状和排列。

（2）细胞核。

（3）细胞质。

单层柱
状上皮

（三）单层柱状上皮

1．染色　　HE。

（1）低倍镜：

1）观察部位在胃的内表面。

2）可见许多小凹陷，凹陷表面覆盖有单层柱状上皮。

（2）高倍镜：

1）细胞为高柱状，排列紧密。

2）细胞核长椭圆形，位于细胞基底部，长轴与细胞长轴平行。

3）近细胞核处胞质呈淡粉红色，核上方胞质空泡状。

4）无杯状细胞。

2．要求识别

（1）上皮细胞的形状和排列。

（2）细胞核。

（3）细胞质。

假复层纤
毛柱状上皮

（四）假复层纤毛柱状上皮

1．染色　　HE。

（1）低倍镜：

1）观察部位在气管的内表面。

2）细胞核呈多层排列。

3）细胞皆与基膜相连。

（2）高倍镜：

1）上皮细胞形态各异，分界不清。游离面可见纤毛。

2）细胞核有3～4层，核的形状、大小、位置各不相同。

3）可见杯状细胞，细胞形似高脚酒杯，顶部膨大，空泡状；细胞核为三角形，近基底部。

4）基膜明显，粉红色，均质状。

2．要求识别

（1）纤毛。

（2）上皮细胞的核和细胞质。

（3）杯状细胞。

（4）基膜。

复层扁
平上皮

（五）复层扁平上皮

1. 染色　　HE。

（1）低倍镜：

1）观察部位在食管的内表面。

2）可见上皮较厚,与深部结缔组织的连接面凹凸不平;由基底面至游离面,细胞逐渐变扁。

（2）高倍镜：

1）由基底面向游离面逐层观察。

2）靠近基膜的一层细胞呈矮柱状或立方形,细胞核圆,位于中央。

3）中间层为数层多边形细胞,核圆形,位于细胞中央。

4）浅层细胞逐渐变扁,游离面细胞扁平,仍可见细胞核。

2. 要求识别

（1）上皮细胞的形状和排列。

（2）细胞核。

（3）细胞质。

变移上皮

（六）变移上皮

1. 染色　　HE。

（1）低倍镜：

1）观察部位在膀胱的内表面。

2）可见膀胱内表面凹凸不平,因收缩形成许多皱襞,上皮较厚,由多层细胞组成,与深部结缔组织间连接面平坦。

（2）高倍镜：

1）由基底面向游离面逐层观察。

2）基底层细胞核圆形或椭圆形,细胞境界不清。

3）中层细胞多边形,核圆。

4）表面细胞为大的多边形,核圆形或椭圆形,位于细胞中央,有的细胞含双核。游离面细胞膜增厚。

2. 要求识别

（1）上皮细胞的形状和排列。

（2）细胞核。

（3）细胞质。

二、复习思考题

（1）单层扁平上皮有何特点?

（2）如何区别单层扁平上皮和复层扁平上皮?

（3）如何鉴别单层柱状上皮和假复层柱状上皮?

（4）光镜下复层扁平上皮和变移上皮有何不同?

三、图 片 思 考 题

图 2-1   图 2-2   图 2-3

（李 颖 傅 奕）

Chapter 2

EPITHELIAL TISSUE

Learning Points

☞ The general structure and classification of epithelial tissues.

☞ The structure and function of the covering epithelium.

☞ The specializations and function of the epithelial cell surfaces.

☞ The definition of the glandular epithelium and gland.

☞ The definition of the exocrine gland and endocrine gland.

Part I   Experiment Contents

simple
squamous
epithelium

1. Simple squamous epithelium

A. Staining   HE.

(1) Low power:

1) The outer surface of the spleen is observed.

2) A layer of flattened cells lines up in order and the mucleus are purplish blue in color.

(2) High power:

1) The cell is flattened.

2) The cytoplasm is extremely thin except where the nucleus exists.

3) The nucleus is flattened, and the long axis is parallel to the main axis of the cell.

B. Identification requirements

(1) Shape and arrangement of the cell body.

(2) Cellular nucleus.

(3) Cytoplasm.

simple
cuboidal
epithelium

2. Simple cuboidal epithelium

A. Staining   HE.

(1) Low power:

1) The epithelium of renal tuble in kindey medulla is observed.

2) Many cross sections of renal tubule are found, and their cavities

are lined by simple cuboidal epithelium.

(2) High power:

1) The cell is cuboidal in shape.

2) The cytoplasm of the cell is stained pale pink.

3) The nucleus of each cell is round in shape and always in the center of the cell.

B. Identification requirements

(1) Shape and arrangement of the cell body.

(2) Cellular nucleus.

(3) Cytoplasm.

simple
columnar
epithelium

3. Simple columnar epithelium

A. Staining　　HE.

(1) Low power:

1) The inner surface of stomach is observed.

2) Many small pits can be found with their surfaces lined by simple columnar epithelium.

(2) High power:

1) The cells are tall columnar and arranged tightly.

2) The nucleus is ovoid in shape, located at the basal part of cell, and its long axis is parallel to the main axis of the cell.

3) The cytoplasm surrounding the nucleus is pale pink in color and vacuolated above the nucleus.

4) No goblet cell can be found.

B. Identification requirements

(1) Shape and arrangement of the cell body.

(2) Cellular nucleus.

(3) Cytoplasm.

pseudostratified
ciliated
columnar
epithelium

4. Pseudostratified ciliated columnar epithelium

A. Staining　　HE.

(1) Low power:

1) The inner surface of trachea is observed.

2) The nuclei are at different levels giving the appearance of stratification.

3) All the cells rest on the basement membrane.

(2) High power:

1) The cells are ciliated on their free surface, different in shape without distinct boundary.

2) 3 to 4 layers of nuclei vary in shape, size, and location.

3）Goblet cell is goblet-like in shape，with a dilatant cell top and a triangular shaped basal situated nucleus.

4）The basement membrane is distinct，homogenous and pale pink in color.

B. Identification requirements

（1）Cilia.

（2）Cellular nucleus and cytoplasm.

（3）Goblet cell.

（4）Basement membrane.

stratified squamous epithelium

5. Stratified squamous epithelium

A. Staining   HE.

（1）Low power：

1）The inner surface of esophagus is observed.

2）The epithelium is thicker，and has a wavy boundary with the underlying connective tissue. The cells become more and more flattened from basal surface to free surface.

（2）High power：

1）The tissue should be observed from the basal surface to the free surface.

2）The basal cells are cuboidal or low columnar with round nuclei located in the centre.

3）The mid-layer is formed by several layers of polygonal cells with round nuclei located in the centre.

4）The superficial cells，with nuclei clearly visible，become more and more flattened.

B. Identification requirements

（1）Shape and arrangement of the cell body.

（2）Nucleus.

（3）Cytoplasm.

transitional epithelium

6. Transitional epithelium

A. Staining   HE.

（1）Low power：

1）The inner surface of urinary bladder is observed.

2）The inner surface of urinary bladder is uneven and forms many rugae with shrinkage. The transitional epithelium is thicker and formed by several layers of cells.

（2）High power：

1）Observe the epithelium from the basal surface to the free surface.

2）The basal cell，with a round or ovoid nucleus，has no distinct boundary.

3）The intermediate cell is polygonal in shape with a round nucleus.

4）The surface cell is large, polygond in shape, with one or two round or ovoid nucleus located in the centre.

B. Identification requirements

（1）Shape and arrangement of the cell body.

（2）Nucleus.

（3）Cytoplasm.

Part II   Questions for Review

（1）What are the characteristics of the simple squamous epithelium?

（2）How to distinguish the difference between the simple squamous epithelium and the stratified squamous epithelium?

（3）How to distinguish the difference between the simple columnar epithelium and the pseudostratified ciliated columnar epithelium?

（4）What are the difference between the stratified squamous epithelium and the transitional epithelium under the light microscope?

Part III   Pictures Questions for Review

Fig.2 - 1   Fig.2 - 2   Fig.2 - 3

（Li Ying, Fu Yi）

第三章

结 缔 组 织

学习要点

☞ 结缔组织的结构特点及分类。
☞ 疏松结缔组织中细胞和纤维的结构和功能。
☞ 疏松结缔组织中基质的组成、特性及功能。
☞ 致密结缔组织、脂肪组织及网状组织的结构和功能。

一、实 验 内 容

（一）疏松结缔组织

1. 染色　台盼蓝活体注射，Verhoeff 碘铁苏木素-伊红染色。

（1）低倍镜：

1）观察部位选择细胞散在、纤维疏松的区域。

2）淡红色纤维与蓝黑色纤维交织成网，纤维间可见细胞核散在分布。

（2）高倍镜：

1）胶原纤维呈淡红色，粗细不等，波浪状行走。

2）弹性纤维为蓝黑色，细，多直行，有分支，末端卷曲。

3）成纤维细胞：胞质丰富，弱嗜碱性，细胞轮廓不清；细胞核大，卵圆形，有时可见明显核仁。

4）巨噬细胞：细胞轮廓清，形态不规则，有突起，胞质嗜酸性，可见蓝色吞噬颗粒；细胞核小，圆形或肾形，染色深。

2. 要求识别

（1）胶原纤维。

（2）弹性纤维。

（3）成纤维细胞。

（4）巨噬细胞。

（二）致密结缔组织

1. 染色　　HE。

（1）低倍镜：

疏松结缔组织

致密结缔组织

1) 粗大的淡红色纤维束平行排列。

2) 束间夹有染成蓝紫色的扁平状细胞核。

（2）高倍镜：

1) 胶原纤维束密集平行排列。

2) 纤维束之间有腱细胞，细胞核长而着色深，沿着纤维束的长轴平行排列，细胞质少而不清。

3) 肌腱外有薄层结缔组织。

2. 要求识别

（1）胶原纤维束的排列。

（2）腱细胞核。

（3）肌腱表面薄层结缔组织。

脂肪组织

（三）脂肪组织

1. 染色　　HE。

（1）低倍镜：

1) 由大量脂肪细胞组成，细胞呈空泡状。

2) 少量疏松结缔组织将脂肪细胞分成不规则小叶。

（2）高倍镜：

1) 脂肪细胞呈圆形或多边形。

2) 胞质中的脂滴在制片过程中被溶解，呈空泡状。胞质弱嗜碱性，被挤成一薄层，位于细胞周边。

3) 细胞核新月形，位于细胞边缘。

4) 可见其他结缔组织的细胞核。

2. 要求识别

（1）脂肪细胞的形状。

（2）脂肪细胞核的形状和位置。

（3）脂肪组织的结构。

网状组织

（四）网状组织

1. 染色　　硝酸银染色。

（1）低倍镜：

1) 网状纤维呈黑色细网状。

2) 细胞核呈黑褐色，细胞其他结构不清。

（2）高倍镜：

1) 网状纤维染成黑色，分支多，相互连接成网。

2) 网状细胞为星形多突起；核卵圆形，染色浅；胞质淡黄色，细胞境界不清。

3) 网状纤维和细胞之间的空白区为基质所在部位。

2. 要求识别

（1）网状细胞。

(2) 网状纤维。

二、复习思考题

(1) 疏松结缔组织的主要组成细胞有哪些？有何形态结构特点？

(2) 疏松结缔组织中三种纤维有何不同？形态结构如何？

(3) 致密结缔组织、脂肪组织及网状组织各有何形态结构特点？

三、图片思考题

图 3 - 1   图 3 - 2   图 3 - 3

（余水长　李　芳）

Chapter 3

CONNECTIVE TISSUE

Learning Points

☞ Structural characteristics and classification of the connective tissues.
☞ Structure and function of the loose connective tissue cells and fibers.
☞ Composition, characteristics and function of the loose connective tissue matrix.
☞ Structure and function of the dense connective tissue, adipose tissue and reticular structure.

Part I   Experiment Contents

loose connective tissue

1. Loose connective tissue

A. Staining   Intravital injection of Trypan blue, the Verhoeff iodine iron hematoxylin-eosin staining.

(1) Low power:

1) Select the area where the cells and the fibers are scattered to observe.

2) The pink fibers and blue-black fibers interweave each other to form a network, and many nuclei scatter among the fibers.

(2) High power:

1) The pink, different in thickness and wavy walking fibers are collagen fibers.

2) Elastic fibers are blue-black, fine, straight, and branched with curly ends.

3) Fibroblast: cell outline is unclear with rich, weakly basophilic cytoplasm and a large oval nucleus, and sometimes prominent nucleoli can be seen.

4) Macrophage: cell outline is clear, its shape is irregular, a lot of blue engulfed particles are visible in the eosinophilic cytoplasm, and a round or kidney-shaped nucleus is small and dark.

B. Idenfication requirements

(1) Collagen fiber.

（2）Elastic fiber.

（3）Fibroblast.

（4）Macrophage.

dense
connective
tissue

2. Dense connective tissue

A. Staining　　HE.

（1）Low power：

1）Coarse pink fiber bundles are densely packed and run in parallel.

2）Elongated flat nuclei stained purple blue lie between the fiber bundles.

（2）High power：

1）The dense collagen fiber bundles are densely packed and arranged in parallel.

2）Tendon cells lie between the fiber bundles，their elongated dark nucleus is arranged in parallel to the long axis of the fiber bundles，and the cytoplasm is sparse and unclear.

3）A thin layer of connective tissue is running outside the tendon.

B. Idenfication requirements

（1）Arrangement of the collagen fiber bundles.

（2）Nucleus of the tendon cell.

（3）A thin connective tissue outside the tendon.

adipose
tissue

3. Adipose tissue

A. Staining　　HE.

（1）Low power：

1）Adipose tissue consists of a large number of adipose cells，which show vacuolization.

2）A small amount of loose connective tissue separate adipose cells into irregular lobules.

（2）High power：

1）Adipose cells are spherical or polyhedral.

2）Each adipose cell contains a large lipid droplet which is dissolved in the slide preparation and leave a large vacuole. Weakly basophilic cytoplasm is squeezed into a thin layer in the cell periphery.

3）Crescent nucleus is located in the cell periphery.

4）Other connective tissue cell nuclei are visible.

B. Idenfication requirements

（1）The shape of adipose cell.

（2）The shape and position of the nucleus of adipose cell.

（3）The structure of adipose tissue.

reticular
tissue

4. Reticular tissue

A. Staining　　Impregnation with silver nitrate.

(1) Low power:

1) Reticular fibers appear as a black thin mesh.

2) The nucleus is dark brown, and the other structures of the cell are unclear.

(2) High power:

1) Reticular fibers are black, multi-branched and connected to form a network.

2) Reticulocyte is star-shaped with many processes; oval nucleus is pale-stained; the cytoplasm shows pale yellow, and cell outline is unclear.

3) Matrix lies in blank area between the reticular fibers and cells.

B. Idenfication requirements

(1) Reticulocyte.

(2) Reticular fiber.

Part II　Questions for Review

(1) What are the major component cells of the loose connective tissue? What are their morphological characteristics?

(2) What are the difference among the three fibers? What are their characteristics?

(3) What are the characteristics of dense connective tissue, adipose tissue and reticular tissue?

Part III　Pictures Questions for Review

Fig.3 - 1

Fig.3 - 2

Fig.3 - 3

(Yu Shuichang, Li Fang)

第四章

软 骨 和 骨

学习要点

☞ 透明软骨、弹性软骨与纤维软骨的结构、生长方式及功能。

☞ 骨组织的结构及其发生的基本过程。

☞ 长骨的结构。

☞ 骨松质与骨密质的结构,骨膜的结构和功能。

一、实 验 内 容

透明软骨

（一）透明软骨

1. 染色　　HE。

（1）低倍镜:

1）从软骨表面逐步向深部观察,注意软骨的一般结构及其在生长过程中的变化。

2）软骨周围有一层染成红色的较致密的结缔组织,即软骨膜。

3）软骨基质的染色深浅不一,从周边部的淡红色到中心部的蓝紫色。

4）软骨陷窝及位于其中的软骨细胞单个或成群分布。

（2）高倍镜:

1）在软骨边缘区为幼稚的软骨细胞,胞体较小,呈扁圆形,其长轴与软骨表面相平行,常单个分布。靠近软骨中心,软骨细胞逐渐增大,为卵圆形、圆形、半圆形或不规则形,常三五成群分布。

2）软骨细胞的核小,圆形或卵圆形,着色深。生活状态时软骨细胞充满整个软骨陷窝。在制片过程中,软骨细胞常皱缩,胞质中的脂滴和糖原被溶解,故胞质中可见大小不一的空泡,而且胞体与软骨囊之间出现空隙。有时整个软骨细胞因制片而脱落,只见空白的软骨陷窝。

3）软骨陷窝周围染成蓝紫色的薄层基质称软骨囊。

4）基质中含少量胶原纤维,排列不规则,折光率几乎与基质相同,无法识别。

2. 要求识别

（1）软骨膜。

（2）软骨陷窝。

（3）软骨细胞。

（4）同源细胞群。

（5）软骨囊。

（6）软骨基质。

骨磨片

（二）骨磨片

1. 染色　　大丽紫。

（1）低倍镜：

1）骨细胞及骨膜、血管、神经和骨髓等软组织已经被去除,故骨磨片上无法观察。

2）骨磨片上散在分布着许多圆形或卵圆形孔洞,大小不等,其中充满色素,为骨单位中央管的横切面,周围有 4～20 层同心圆排列的骨板。外缘可见一条折光较强的轮廓线,即黏合线。

3）在骨单位之间可见若干层平行排列的骨板,且无中央管构成的间骨板,形状不规则。

4）骨陷窝位于骨板内或骨板之间,为扁椭圆形,其分布与骨板走向一致。骨陷窝的周围发出许多细长的线条,为骨小管,相邻骨陷窝的骨小管彼此连通。在骨单位内,骨小管的走向大都与中央管长轴垂直,以此为中心向周围辐射,但不超越该骨单位的黏合线。

（2）高倍镜：骨磨片较厚,不宜使用高倍镜观察。

2. 要求识别

（1）骨单位。

（2）间骨板。

（3）骨陷窝。

（4）骨小管。

二、复习思考题

（1）简述各种骨细胞的结构和功能。

（2）名词解释：骨单位、同源细胞群。

三、图片思考题

图 4-1　　　　　　图 4-2　　　　　　图 4-3

（李　芳　余水长）

Chapter 4

CARTILAGE AND BONE

Learning Points

☞ The structure, growth pattern and function of the hyaline cartilage, elastic cartilage and fibrocartilage.

☞ The structure of bone tissue and the basic process of ossification.

☞ The structure of long bone.

☞ The structure of compact bone, spongy bone, and the structure and function of periosteum.

Part I   Experiment Contents

hyaline cartilage

1. Hyaline cartilage

A. Staining   HE.

(1) Low power:

1) Gradually observe the cartilage from the surface to the deep, and pay attention to the general structure of the cartilage and its changes during its growth.

2) Perichondrium, a layer of dense connective tissue stained red, covers the surface of the cartilage.

3) Cartilage matrix stain varies from light red in the periphery to the purple blue in the center.

4) The cartilage lacunae and the chondrocytes in cartilage matrix are distributed either individually or in a group.

(2) High power:

1) At the periphery of the cartilage, young chondrocytes have a spindle or elliptical shape, with the long axis parallel to the surface. In the deeper part of the cartilage, cells are more mature and round, and often gathered in groups.

2) The nucleus of chondrocyte is small, round or oval, stained dark. In living tissue, the chondrocytes fill the lacunae completely, but in histological preparations, both the cells and the matrix shrink, showing gaps between chondrocytes and cartilage capsule, and the chondrocyte falling off leaving the empty cartilage lacunae clear

visible. The cytoplasmic lipid droplets and glycogen are dissolved, resulting in vacuolation in cytoplasm.

3) The thin-layer matrix surrounding the cartilage lacuna is called cartilage capsule stained in dark blue.

4) The cartilage matrix contains a few collagen fibrils, which are irregularly arranged and indiscernible because of the same refractive index with the ground substance in which they are embedded.

B. Identification requirements

(1) Perichondrium.

(2) Cartilage lacuna.

(3) Chondrocyte.

(4) Isogenous group.

(5) Cartilage capsule.

(6) Cartilage matrix.

ground
bone slide

2. Ground bone slide

A. Staining   Dahlia violet.

(1) Low power:

1) Osteacytes, periosteum, blood vessels, nerves and bone marrow can not be observed as been removed.

2) Round or oval holes of varying sizes, filled with pigment, are the central canal of the osteons, and for each of them 4 to 20 concentric lamellae of bone matrix are found, and a obvious bright line, bone cement line, is found covering the outer edge of each osteon.

3) Interstitial lamellae are irregularly shaped groups of parallel lamellae disposing between the osteons.

4) Osseous lacuna is oval in shape and distributes in or between osseous lamellae, bone canaliculi, small tubules send out from one lacuna and connect with the bone canaliculi from other lacuna. Within each osteon bone canaliculi are perpendicular to the surface of the central canal, extend radially from it but not exceed the cement line.

(2) High power: High magnification is not suitable because the ground bone slide is rather thick.

B. Identification requirements

(1) Osteon.

(2) Interstitial lamellae.

(3) Osseous lacuna.

(4) Bone canaliculus.

Part II   Questions for Review

(1) Briefly describe the structure and function of various types of cells in the

osseous tissue.

（2）Provide an explanation for the following terms：osteon，isogenous group.

Part III   Pictures Questions for Review

Fig.4 - 1   Fig.4 - 2   Fig.4 - 3

（Li Fang，Yu Shuichang）

第五章

血　液

学习要点

☞ 血液的组成及各类血细胞的结构特点、功能和正常值。

☞ 造血干细胞、造血祖细胞的基本概念。

☞ 红细胞系,粒细胞系,单核细胞系的发生阶段及变化规律。

☞ 巨核细胞系的发生与血小板的生成。

一、实 验 内 容

（一）血涂片

血涂片

1. 血涂片的制作

采血:采血部位为无名指,70%的乙醇消毒,采血针迅速刺入皮肤,擦去第一滴血。以洁净载玻片承接血滴,血滴位于距载玻片一端 1 cm 处,直径约3 mm,注意载玻片不接触皮肤。

涂片:左手平托载玻片,右手取另一载玻片紧密接触血滴,两载玻片夹角为30°～45°,待血滴散开呈一条线时,将右手载玻片在左手载玻片上平稳推向前方,形成血膜。血膜厚度以能看到载玻片下方字迹为宜,末端呈舌形为佳,待其自然干燥。

染色:取干燥的血涂片,以蜡笔或蜡块划出染色区,先滴加 Wright 染液至恰好布满染色区,染色约 3 min;再滴加等量磷酸缓冲液,轻轻吹动,使其与染液充分混合,等待 5 min后,用自来水轻洗后竖直放置,待其自然干燥。

（1）低倍镜:

1）血细胞均匀分布,分散无重叠。

2）红细胞呈橘红色。

3）白细胞核呈蓝紫色。

（2）高倍镜:

1）红细胞:数量多,直径约为 7.5 μm,双凹圆盘状,无细胞核,胞质呈橘红色,中央染色浅,周围染色深。

2）中性粒细胞:白细胞中占比最大,占白细胞总数的50%～70%,细胞圆形,直径为10～12 μm,细胞核紫蓝色分为2～5 叶,以 3 叶居多,叶间以细丝相连,细胞质呈粉红色,内含许多细小而均匀的淡紫红色颗粒。

3）淋巴细胞:占白细胞总数的20%～30%,细胞呈圆形,大小不一,其中直径为 6～

8 μm的小淋巴细胞占大部分,小淋巴细胞核为圆形或椭圆形,染色深,一侧有浅凹;细胞质少,染成天蓝色,胞质内可见少量嗜天青颗粒。

4)单核细胞:占白细胞总数的 3%～8%,细胞呈圆形,直径 14～20 μm,是最大的白细胞。细胞核大,肾形或马蹄铁形,细胞质较淋巴细胞丰富,为浅灰色,含有细小的嗜天青颗粒。

5)嗜酸性粒细胞:占白细胞总数的 0.5%～3%,细胞呈圆形,直径 10～15 μm,核分两叶、以细丝相连;胞质浅粉红色,内含许多粗大而均匀的鲜红色圆形颗粒。

6)嗜碱性粒细胞:占白细胞总数的 0～1%,不易找到。细胞呈圆形,直径 10～12 μm,核呈"S"形或不规则形,着色浅;胞质内含大小不等、分布不均的深蓝紫色嗜碱性颗粒;细胞核常因被颗粒覆盖而显示不清。

7)血小板:常聚集成群,每个血小板状如蓝紫色碎片,直径 2～4 μm,形态不规则,中央部分可见深色的颗粒。

2.要求识别

(1)红细胞。

(2)中性粒细胞。

(3)淋巴细胞。

(4)单核细胞。

(5)血小板。

网织红细胞

(二)网织红细胞

1.染色　　煌焦油蓝染色法。

(1)低倍镜:

1)选择血细胞分布均匀、无重叠的区域进行观察。

2)红细胞呈橘红色,白细胞核呈蓝紫色。

(2)高倍镜:

1)网织红细胞体积略大于红细胞。

2)网织红细胞胞质内可见蓝色物质,呈网状或细颗粒状。

2.要求识别　　网织红细胞。

二、复 习 思 考 题

简述白细胞、红细胞的结构特点和功能。

三、图 片 思 考 题

图 5-1　　　　　　图 5-2　　　　　　图 5-3　　　　　　图 5-4

(岳海源　郑　英)

Chapter 5

BLOOD

Learning Points

- ☞ The blood composition, the structure, function and normal count of various types of blood cells.
- ☞ The basic concept of hematopoietic stem cells and hematopoietic progenitor cells.
- ☞ Maturational stages and morphological changes of erythrocytic series, granulocytic series and monocytic series.
- ☞ The development of megakaryocytic series and the formation of platelets.

Part I Experiment Contents

blood
smear

1. Blood smear

A. Blood smear preparation

Blood taking: Firstly, sterilize the distal of ring finger with 70% ethanol. Then quickly penetrate blood taking needle into the skin of finger tip, wipe away the first drop of blood and place a small drop of blood approximately 3 mm in diameter on the surface of a clean glass slide at a distance of 1 cm from the end, avoiding contacting with finger skin.

Smear producing: Hold the slide with the blood drop in the left hand, and use the spreader in the right hand to contact the blood drop. The approximate angle between the two slides is 30 to 45 degrees. When the slide edge touches the blood drop, the blood spread along the edge. Then push the spreader slide to the left in a smooth, quick motion. The smear should cover approximately half the slide with a gradual transition from thick to thin. No ridges should be present and the end (called the "tongue edge") should be smooth and even. In the tongue edge the red blood cells should not be routinely overlapped. Wait until the smear is completely air-dried.

Smear staining: When the smear is completely dried, draw the staining area with a mark pen, drop a layer of Wright stain on the surface of the slide, wait about 3 minutes, and then add the same amount phosphate buffer, gently blow, and make sure the solutions are fully mixed, wait about 5 minutes, after washing with tap water, place the slide vertically, allowing slide to dry completely.

(1) Low power:

1) The blood cells are evenly spread out not overlapping each other.

2) Erythrocytes are reddish-orange.

3) Leukocyte nuclei are purple blue.

(2) High power:

1) Erythrocytes: Most of the cells are erythrocytes or red blood cells. They are biconcave discs approximately 7.5 μm in diameter, without nuclei. The cytoplasm is stained reddish orange, the central part stained lightly while periphery darker.

2) Neutrophils: The largest percentage of leukocytes or white blood cells accounts for 50% to 70% of the total number of leukocytes. They are round in shape and 10 to 12 μm in diameter. They have nuclei that are stained purple blue. Many of them have segmented nuclei, meaning that the nucleus is pinched into two to five smaller parts that are still connected to each other by thin thread. Three lobes are most likely to be seen. The cytoplasm is pink and contains many small and uniform granules stained reddish-orange.

3) Lymphocytes: They take up for 20% to 30% of total number of leukocytes. They are round in shape and have different sizes. Most of them are small lymphocytes which are 6 to 8 μm in diameter. The nucleus of small lymphocyte is round or oval, intensely stained and sometime with a dimple; the cytoplasm is less, stained sky-blue and contains a few azurophilic granules.

4) Monocytes: They are usually the largest leukocytes present. They take up 3%~8% of total number of leukocytes. They are round in shape and 14 to 20 μm in diameter. The nucleus is large, kidney or horseshoe shaped. The cytoplasm is more abundant than in lymphocytes and has a greyish blue with very fine azurophilic granules.

5) Eosinophils: They number for 0.5% to 3% of total leukocytes. They are round in shape and 10 to 15 μm in diameter. The nucleus is pinched into two lobes that are still connected by thin thread. Cytoplasm is pinkish, containing many bulky, and uniform and spherical bright red granules.

6) Basophils: They number only for 0 to 1% of total number of leukocytes and therefore it is difficult to find. They are round in shape and 10 to 12 μm in diameter. The nucleus shows "S" shape or irregular shape, lightly stained. Cytoplasm includes unevenly distributed dark purple blue basophilic granules which appear irregular in size and shape. The nucleus is often covered by granules and the display is not clear.

7) Platelets: They often appear in clumps, each platelet looks like a purple blue small fragment which is 2 to 4 μm in diameter, irregular in shape and contains dark stained granules in the central part.

B. Identification requirements

（1）Erythrocyte.

（2）Neutrophil.

（3）Lymphocyte.

（4）Monocyte.

（5）Platelet.

2. Reticulocyte

A. Staining   Brilliant cresyl blue staining.

（1）Low power：

1）Look for part of the slide where the cells are distributed

reticulocyte   uniformly and in a single layer.

2）Erythrocytes are red-orange. Leukocyte nuclei are purple blue.

（2）High power：

1）Reticulocyte is slightly larger than erythrocyte.

2）Blue materials with the shape of mesh or fine particles can be seen in the cytoplasm of reticulocyte.

B. Identification requirements   Reticulocyte.

Part II   Questions for Review

Briefly describe the structural features and functions of erythrocyte and leukocytes.

Part III   Pictures Questions for Review

Fig.5 - 1   Fig.5 - 2   Fig.5 - 3   Fig.5 - 4

(Yue Haiyuan，Zheng Ying)

第六章

肌 组 织

学习要点

☞ 肌组织的特性。

☞ 骨骼肌的光镜结构,电镜结构和功能。

☞ 心肌的光镜结构,电镜结构和功能。

☞ 平滑肌的光镜结构和功能。

一、实 验 内 容

骨骼肌

(一) 骨骼肌

1. 染色 　 HE。

(1) 低倍镜:

1) 在纵切面上,骨骼肌纤维呈细长纤维状,平行排列,肌纤维之间有少量结缔组织,即肌内膜。

2) 每条肌纤维中有许多细胞核,位于细胞周缘。

3) 肌纤维横切面呈圆形或多边形。

(2) 高倍镜:

1) 骨骼肌的纵切面上可见明暗相间的周期性横纹,即明带和暗带,明带中间有一条暗线横过,即 Z 线。暗带中间有一条染色较浅的窄带,称 H 带,中间有一条暗线,称 M 线。

2) 在肌纤维的周缘靠近肌膜的地方,可见多个扁平的细胞核。

3) 肌纤维横断面圆形或多边形,其内的肌原纤维呈点状。

2. 要求识别

(1) 肌细胞核。

(2) 横纹。

(3) 明带和暗带。

心肌

(二) 心肌

1. 染色 　 HE。

(1) 低倍镜:

1) 心肌纵切面呈矮柱状,有分支,并与邻近的细胞相连接。

2) 心肌细胞核 1～2 个,位于肌纤维中央。

3）心肌横断面呈圆形，多边形或不规则形，大小不一。

（2）高倍镜：

1）纵切面上，心肌细胞核呈椭圆形，长轴和肌纤维长轴一致，位于肌纤维中部。

2）心肌纤维有横纹，但不如骨骼肌明显。

3）在心肌细胞连接处，为着色较深的细线，称闰盘。

4）横断面上，心肌细胞核呈圆形或卵圆形，位于心肌细胞的中央。

5）切片中有许多不规则的心肌纤维斜切面。

2．要求识别

（1）肌细胞核。

（2）横纹。

（3）闰盘。

平滑肌

（三）平滑肌

1．染色　　HE。

（1）低倍镜：

1）纵切面肌纤维呈长梭形，彼此平行排列，细胞核呈椭圆形或杆状位于肌纤维中央，少量疏松结缔组织散在于肌束之间。

2）横断面上肌纤维大小不等，粉红色，可见不同程度的斜切面。

（2）高倍镜：

1）纵切面上，平滑肌纤维为长梭形，两端尖细，中间较粗，细胞质染成粉红色。

2）平滑肌细胞含有一个椭圆形或长杆状的细胞核，居中。当肌纤维处于收缩状态时，细胞核可呈螺旋形扭曲。

3）平滑肌纤维的粗部和相邻的平滑肌纤维的细部相间排列。

4）横断面呈圆形或不规则形，大小不一。在大的断面含有位居中央的核，在小的断面没有细胞核。

2．要求识别

（1）肌细胞核。

（2）平滑肌纤维的排列。

二、复习思考题

（1）比较三种肌组织的光镜结构特点。

（2）骨骼肌和心肌的超微结构有哪些不同特点？

三、图片思考题

图6-1　　　　　图6-2　　　　　图6-3

（岳海源　郑　英）

Chapter 6

MUSCLE TISSUE

Learning Points

☞ Features of muscle tissue.

☞ The structure of skeletal muscle under light microscope and electron microscope and its related function.

☞ The structure of cardiac muscle under light microscope and electron microscope and its related function.

☞ The structure of smooth muscle under light microscope and its related function.

Part I   Experiment Contents

skeletal
muscle

1. Skeletal muscle

A. Staining   HE.

(1) Low power:

1) On the longitudinal section, skeletal muscle fibers are long cylindrical striated cells arranged in parallel to each other. The delicate connective tissue covering the surface of each fiber is the endomysium.

2) Each skeletal muscle fiber contains many nuclei which are peripherally located just under the sarcolemma.

3) On the cross section, the skeletal muscle fibers show round or polygonal profiles.

(2) High power:

1) On the longitudinal section, the cross-striations with alternating light and dark bands are obvious, a dark line cross the light band is Z line, and in the middle of the dark band a narrow lightly stained band is the H band, within which a dark line is M line.

2) Many flattened nuclei are peripherally located in the skeletal muscle fiber just under the sarcolemma.

3) On the cross section, the skeletal muscle fibers show round or polygonal profiles, and within each profile the myofibrils give a stippled appearance.

B. Identification requirements

(1) Nuclei of skeletal muscle fiber.

(2) Cross-striations.

(3) Light and dark bands.

2. Cardiac muscle

cardiac
muscle

A. Staining   HE.

(1) Low power:

1) On the longitudinal section, the cardiac muscle fibers are short cylindrical and may branch at their ends to form connections with adjacent cells.

2) Each cardiac muscle fiber possesses one or two centrally located nuclei.

3) On the cross section, the profile of the cardiac muscle is polygonal or irregular in shape and various in size.

(2) High power:

1) On the longitudinal section, the nucleus is oval and centrally located in the fiber.

2) The cross-striated banding pattern of cardic muscle fiber is identical to that of skeletal muscle fiber but not as clear as that.

3) The dark-staining transverse line that appears in myocardial cell junctions is intercalated disk.

4) On the cross section, the nuclei of cardiac muscle fibers are round or oval and located in the center of the cells.

5) Numerous irregular oblique profiles of cardiac muscle fibers are shown on a cross section.

B. Identification requirements

(1) Nuclei of cardiac muscle fiber.

(2) Cross-striations.

(3) Intercalated disk.

3. Smooth muscle

smooth
muscle

A. Staining   HE.

(1) Low power:

1) On the longitudinal section, smooth muscle fibers are spindle-shaped with an centrally located elongated nucleus and a few loose connective tissue distributes among the smooth muscle bundles.

2) On the cross section, the profiles of smooth muscle fibers are various in size, stained pink and many are their oblique sections.

(2) High power：

1) On the longitudinal section, smooth muscle fibers are largest at their midpoints and taper toward their ends, and their cytoplasm is stained pink.

2) Each smooth muscle fiber contains an oval or elongated nucleus located in the center of the broadest part of the cell. If contraction of the cell has occurred, the nucleus may be folded or coiled.

3) The narrow part of one cell lies adjacent to the broad parts of neighboring cells.

4) On the cross section, the smooth muscle fibers present round or irregularly polygonal profiles with variations in diameter and only the largest profiles contain a centrally placed nucleus. No nucleus is found in the smaller profiles.

B. Identification requirements

(1) Nuclei of smooth muscle fiber.

(2) The arrangement of smooth muscle fibers.

Part II　Questions for Review

(1) Compare the structural characteristics of three types of the muscle tissue under light microscope.

(2) What are the difference in the ultrastructure between cardiac muscle and skeletal muscle?

Part III　Pictures Questions for Review

Fig.6 - 1　　　　　　Fig.6 - 2　　　　　　Fig.6 - 3

(Yue Haiyuan，Zheng Ying)

第七章

神 经 组 织

学习要点

- ☞ 神经组织的基本结构。
- ☞ 神经细胞的光镜与超微结构。
- ☞ 神经细胞的分类。
- ☞ 突触的超微结构。
- ☞ 各种神经胶质细胞的结构和功能特点。
- ☞ 有髓及无髓神经纤维的光镜与超微结构。

一、实 验 内 容

运动
神经元

（一）运动神经元

1. 染色　　HE。

（1）低倍镜：

1）在脊髓横切面中部首先找到中央管及周围的灰质,灰质呈蝴蝶形。灰质腹侧较粗短的部分为前角,在前角中可见到一些多边形细胞,大小不一,为运动神经元的胞体。

2）胞体内可见大而圆的细胞核。

3）胞体周围有少数较短的突起。

（2）高倍镜：

1）多极神经元的细胞核大,圆形,居中,着色浅,核仁明显。

2）多极神经元通常突起很多,但在切片上仅见少数较短的突起,大多为树突。

3）细胞质内充满蓝紫色块状或斑状的嗜染质,又称尼氏体。核周和树突的胞质内均可见尼氏体;轴突中无尼氏体,起始部呈圆锥状,着色浅,称轴丘。借此可区分树突和轴突。

4）切片中可见神经胶质细胞,胞质呈中性,不着色,仅见细胞核,大小不等,圆形或卵圆形,着色浅,可见核仁。

2. 要求识别

（1）多极神经元。

（2）细胞核。

（3）尼氏体。

（4）树突和轴突。

有髓神经
纤维横断面

（二）有髓神经纤维（横断面）

1. 染色   HE。

（1）低倍镜：

1）整个神经外面包以疏松结缔组织，称神经外膜，其中有成群的脂肪细胞和小血管。

2）神经外膜伸入神经内形成神经束膜，将神经分成大小不等的神经束。神经束膜纤维较多，其内层有多层扁平上皮细胞构成神经束上皮。

3）神经束膜伸入神经束内，分布在每一根神经纤维的周围，称神经内膜。

（2）高倍镜：

1）有髓神经纤维的横断面呈圆形，大小不等。

2）神经纤维中央紫红色的圆点为轴突的横断面，轴突周围为髓鞘，着色淡，呈淡红色网格状。

3）有的断面周缘可见染成紫蓝色的施万细胞核。

2. 要求识别

（1）轴突。

（2）髓鞘。

（3）神经内膜。

（4）神经束膜。

（5）神经外膜。

有髓神经
纤维纵切面

（三）有髓神经纤维（纵切面）

1. 染色   HE。

（1）低倍镜：

1）神经纤维沿纵向紧密排列成束。

2）整条神经外面有结缔组织构成的神经外膜，浅红色，其中含有小血管及脂肪细胞。

3）神经束膜及神经内膜不易分辨。

（2）高倍镜：

1）神经纤维排列紧密，在神经纤维中央有一条深蓝色的细线为轴突。

2）轴突周围是髓鞘，制片时脂类被溶解而剩下淡红色的蛋白质网状结构。

3）髓鞘边缘常可见长杆状的施万细胞核。

4）相邻的施万细胞间不完全连接，形成缩窄处，称郎飞结。

2. 要求识别

（1）轴突。

（2）髓鞘。

（3）施万细胞核。

（4）郎飞结。

运动终板

（四）运动终板

1.染色　氯化金。

（1）低倍镜：

1）可见许多被分离的骨骼肌纤维，平行排列，肌细胞核未被染色。

2）运动神经元的轴突终末部分被染成黑色，分支附着在骨骼肌纤维表面。

（2）高倍镜：

1）骨骼肌纤维可见明暗交替的周期性横纹。

2）轴突分支末端呈纽扣状或葡萄样膨大，附着于骨骼肌纤维表面。

2.要求识别

（1）肌纤维。

（2）横纹。

（3）运动终板。

二、复习思考题

（1）简述神经元的超微结构特点。

（2）比较树突和轴突的不同特点。

（3）简述神经胶质细胞的结构特点。

（4）简述神经末梢的结构特点。

三、图片思考题

图 7-1

图 7-2

图 7-3

图 7-4

（陈　雪　郭　辉）

Chapter 7

NERVE TISSUE

Learning Points

☞ The basic structure of the nerve tissue.

☞ The structure and ultrastructure of the nerve cell.

☞ The classification of nerve cells.

☞ The ultrastructure of the synapse.

☞ The structural and functional characteristics of different types of glial cells.

☞ The structure and ultrastructure of myelinated and non-myelinated nerve fibers.

Part I   Experiment Contents

motor
neuron

1. Motor neuron

A. Staining   HE.

(1) Low power:

1) On the cross section, the spinal cord central canal and the butterfly-shaped gray matter around it are located. The dumpy anterior horn of the gray matter is identified at its ventral part, in which the polygonal cells, the bodies of motor neurons, are found and these cells are various in size.

2) A big and round nucleus is located in the center of the neuron.

3) Many short processes extend from the cell body.

(2) High power:

1) The nuclei of multipolar neurons are large, round, lightly stained, and centrally located, with its prominent nucleolus.

2) The multipolar neurons possess numerous processes, and a few of which seen on the same section are most dendrites. but most of them are dendrites.

3) Accumulations of basophilic nucleoprotein (Nissl body) are found distributed in the cell body and dendrites, but not in the axon hillock, the site of the origin of the axon by which dendrites and axon can be differeniated.

4) The cytoplasm of glial cells is neutral, which can't be stained. The nucleus is

round or oval, various in size, and lightly stained. Its nucleolus is prominent.

B. Identification requirements

(1) Multipolar neuron.

(2) Nucleus.

(3) Nissle body.

(4) Dendrites and axon.

myelinated
nerve fibers
(cross section)

2. Myelinated nerve fibers (cross section)

A. Staining   HE.

(1) Low power:

1) The loose connective tissue covering the outer surface of the nerve is the epineurium, among which the adipose cells and small blood vessels can be observed.

2) The epineurium also extends into the nerve, fills the space between the bundles of nerve fibers, and forms perineurium, covering the surface of each bundle of nerve fibers. A layer of flattened epithelium lain on the inner surface of perineurium is called nerve tract epithelium.

3) The connective tissue extending from the perineurium covers the surface of each nerve fiber and forms the structure of endoneurium.

(2) High power:

1) The cross section of each nerve fiber is round in shape and different in size.

2) The darkly stained spot located in the center of each nerve fiber is the cross section of axon. The myelin sheath is around the axon which is stained in the pink mesh-like structure.

3) For some of the nerve fibers, the purple-blue stained nuclei of Schwann cells are distributed peripherally.

B. Identification requirements

(1) Axon.

(2) Myelin sheath.

(3) Endoneurium.

(4) Perineurium.

(5) Epineurium.

myelinated
nerve fibers
(longitudinal
section)

3. Myelinated nerve fibers (longitudinal section)

A. Staining   HE.

(1) Low power:

1) Nerve fibers are closely longitudinally arranged to form bundles.

2) Epineurium, a dense irregular connective tissue layer, surrounds the entire nerve, and simultaneously adipose cells and small blood vessels are also found in it.

3）Endoneurium and perineurium is not easily distinguishable.

（2）High power：

1）Nerve fibers are closely arranged in parallel，and the blue-black line in the central portion of each fiber is axon.

2）Around the axon，the "foamy"，grainy appearance of the myelin sheath is noticed，because the lipid portion of the membranes has been dissolved out during the tissue fixation.

3）Long rod-shaped nuclei of Schwann cells are distributed peripherally around the myelin.

4）The points at which two Schwann cells meet are called nodes of Ranvier. Adjacent Schwann cells are not continuous at the node.

B. Identification requirements

（1）Axon.

（2）Myelin sheath.

（3）Nucleus of Schwann cell.

（4）Nodes of Ranvier.

motor end plate

4. Motor end plate

A. Staining   Gold chloride.

（1）Low power：

1）The skeletal muscle fibers are arranged in parallel，and their nuclei are not stained.

2）The terminal part of the axon of a motor neuron is stained black and divided into several branches which distributed on the surface of skeletal muscle fibers.

（2）High power：

1）The alternating light and dark bands of cross striation are clearly visible on the surface of skeletal muscle fibers.

2）The small terminal branches of the axon form a cluster of small bulbous swellings or grape-like enlargements on the surface of skeletal muscle fibers.

B. Identification requirements

（1）Skeletal muscle fiber.

（2）Cross striation.

（3）Motor end plate.

Part II Questions for Review

（1）Briefly describe the ultrastructural features of neurons.

（2）Compare the different characteristics of dendrites and axons.

（3）Briefly describe the structural features of the glial cells.

（4）Briefly describe the structural features of nerve endings.

Part III   Pictures Questions for Review

Fig.7 - 1

Fig.7 - 2

Fig.7 - 3

Fig.7 - 4

(Chen Xue, Guo Hui)

第八章

循 环 系 统

学习要点

☞ 大、中、小动脉的结构与功能。

☞ 静脉的一般形态结构特点。

☞ 三种毛细血管的形态结构特点。

☞ 心脏壁各层结构与功能。

一、实 验 内 容

中动脉与
大静脉

（一）中动脉与大静脉

1. 染色　　HE。

（1）低倍镜：

1）血管壁由内向外分 3 层，即内膜、中膜和外膜；横断面上动脉腔圆、壁厚，静脉腔大、壁薄。

2）中动脉内膜薄，内皮下层很难辨认，内弹性膜明显。

3）中膜厚，由环形排列的平滑肌纤维围成，平滑肌细胞间可见胶原纤维和弹性纤维。

4）外膜为结缔组织，染色浅，外弹性膜不连续、包含几层，可见营养血管和神经。

5）大静脉内膜薄，内弹性膜不发达。中膜薄，为稀疏分布的环形平滑肌。外膜厚，为结缔组织，没有外弹性膜，可见平滑肌横切面，为纵行平滑肌束。

（2）高倍镜：

1）中动脉内膜表面可见紫蓝色内皮细胞核突出腔面。

2）中动脉中膜由大量的平滑肌纤维及胶原纤维环绕管壁而成，平滑肌纤维之间可见较细而散在的弹性纤维。

2. 要求识别

（1）内膜、内皮、内弹性膜。

（2）中膜、外弹性膜。

（3）外膜。

（二）大动脉

大动脉

1. 染色　　雷索辛复红。

(1) 低倍镜：

1) 大动脉是弹性动脉，管壁由内向外分3层：内膜、中膜和外膜。

2) 中膜最厚，富有弹性纤维，其中夹有少量平滑肌，内弹性膜不明显。

3) 外膜薄，外弹性膜不明显，出现少量血管和神经纤维。

(2) 高倍镜：弹性纤维呈紫色线条环形排列。

2. 要求识别　　弹性膜。

（三）毛细血管

1. 染色　　HE。

(1) 低倍镜：在结缔组织中有许多毛细血管，管腔最细，管径为7～9 μm。

毛细血管

(2) 高倍镜：管壁只有1～2个内皮细胞，细胞核向管腔面突出。

2. 要求识别

(1) 内皮。

(2) 各种断面的毛细血管。

（四）小动脉与小静脉

1. 染色　　HE。

(1) 低倍镜：

1) 小动脉腔小而圆，管壁较厚。

2) 小静脉常与小动脉伴行，腔大壁薄。

小动脉与
小静脉

(2) 高倍镜：

1) 小动脉中膜厚，由环形平滑肌围成，内弹性膜明显，外弹性膜缺如。

2) 小静脉中膜薄，外膜较厚，腔内有血液。

2. 要求识别

(1) 小动脉。

(2) 小静脉。

（五）心脏

1. 染色　　HE。

(1) 低倍镜：

1) 心脏壁由内向外分为：心内膜、心肌膜、心外膜。

2) 心内膜的表面为单层扁平上皮，即内皮，内皮下层为薄层结缔组织及少量平滑肌细胞，内皮下层深部疏松结缔组织为心内膜下层。

心脏

3) 心肌膜厚，可见大量的心肌细胞。

4) 心外膜由结缔组织构成，较疏松，其中可见脂肪细胞、血管、神经，外表面有间皮。

(2) 高倍镜：心内膜下层的结缔组织内可见成群分布的浦肯野纤维（束细胞），细胞体积大，胞质染色浅，核圆居中。

2. 要求识别

(1) 心内膜各层。

(2) 心肌膜。

(3) 心外膜。

(4) 蒲肯野纤维。

心瓣膜

(六) 心瓣膜

1. 染色　　HE。

(1) 低倍镜: 心瓣膜表面有内皮, 内皮下为致密结缔组织。

(2) 高倍镜:

1) 致密结缔组织中胶原纤维染成紫色, 可见深染的成纤维细胞的细胞核。

2) 在心肌附着端根部, 内皮下方可见少量平滑肌肌纤维。

2. 要求识别

(1) 心瓣膜。

(2) 心室面。

(3) 心房面。

二、复习思考题

(1) 简述循环系统的组成。

(2) 简述各型动脉和静脉的结构特点。

(3) 简述毛细血管的分类, 各型毛细血管有何不同。

(4) 简述心壁的构成, 以及心脏传导系统的组成、分布与结构特点。

三、图片思考题

图 8-1

图 8-2

图 8-3

图 8-4

（李冬梅　韩晓冬　丁卫东）

Chapter 8

CIRCULATORY SYSTEM

Learning Points

☞ The structure and function of the large arteries, medium-sized arteries, small arteries.
☞ The general morphological features of the veins.
☞ The morphological features of the three types of capillaries.
☞ The structure and function of the heart walls.

Part I   Experiment Contents

1. Medium-sized arteries and large veins

medium-sized arteries and large veins

A. Staining   HE.

(1) Low power:

1) The walls of blood vessels are composed of three coats: tunica intima, tunica media and tunica adventitia. In cross section, the lumen of an artery is round and has a thicker wall; while the lumen of a vein is larger and has a thinner wall.

2) The tunica intima of the medium-sized artery is thinner and therefore the subendothelial layer is not obvious; however, the internal elastic membrane is well developed.

3) The tunic media is thicker, and consists mainly of circularly arranged smooth muscle fibers. Between muscle cells are fine collagenous fibers and elastic fibers.

4) The tunic adventitia is composed of a layer of loose connective tissue which is refractory to ordinarily staining and the external elastic membrane is divided into several lamellae. The vasa vasorum and small nerves can be observed.

5) The tunic intima of the large veins is thin and its internal elastic membrane is not prominent. It contains relatively thick tunica adventitia and thin tunica media. The tunica media consists of several layers of circularly arranged smooth muscle fibers. The tunica adventitia is composed of relatively well developed connective tissue, in which

the cross sections of quite a number of smooth muscle fibers can easily be seen but the external elastic membrane is invisible.

(2) High power：

1) The purple blue staining nuclei can be seen on the surface of the tunica intima in the medium-sized artery.

2) The tunic media of the medium-sized artery contains a large number of smooth muscle fibers. Between the muscle cells are fine collagenous fibers and elastic fibers.

B. Identification requirements

(1) Tunica intima，endothelium and internal elastic membrane.

(2) Tunica media，external elastic membrane.

(3) Tunica adventitia.

large artery
(aorta)

2. Large artery (aorta)

A. Staining　　Resorcin eosin.

(1) Low power：

1) This is an example of the elastic artery，and three layers—tunica intima，media and adventitia can be distinguished.

2) The tunica media is the thickest and mainly composed of fine elastic fibers. The elastic tissue in the tunica media is well developed，where many elastic membranous layers or lamellar networks alternate with smooth muscle cells.

3) Tunica adventitia is composed mainly of collagenous fibers and some elastic fibers extending out from the outermost layer of the elastic membranes. Also present in the tunica adventitia are small blood vessels and small bundles of nerve fibers.

(2) High power：Elastic fibers are stained purple and circular lines can be identified.

B. Identification requirements　　Elastic membrane.

capillaries

3. Capillaries

A. Staining　　HE.

(1) Low power：Numerous capillaries exist in the connective tissue. These are very small vessels which is 7 to 9 μm in diameter.

(2) High power：The capillary is made up of 1 or 2 endothelial cells. The nuclei of the endothelial cells usually bulge into the lumen of the capillary.

B. Identification requirements

(1) Endothelium.

(2) Different sections of the capillary.

small arteries
and veins

4. Small arteries and veins

A. Staining   HE.

(1) Low power：

1) Small arteries have smaller lumens and thicker walls.

2) Small veins are frequently accompanied closely by small arteries. In contrast, small veins have larger lumens and thinner walls.

(2) High power：

1) The tunica media is relatively thicker and composed of circularly arranged layers of smooth muscle cells. The presence of the distinct inner elastic membrane and the absence of the external elastic membrane should be noticed.

2) The small veins are vessels with much thinner walls and are usually filled with blood. The tunica media is thinner and the tunica adventitia is thicker.

B. Identification requirements

(1) Small arteries.

(2) Small veins.

heart

5. Heart

A. Staining   HE.

(1) Low power：

1) The wall of the heart consists of three layers: an inner endocardium, a middle myocardium and an outer epicardium.

2) The inner surface of the endocardium is lined by a single layer of endothelial cells. Immediately beneath the endothelial cells is the thin subendothelial layer, containing smooth muscle cells. External to this is a thick layer of loose connective tissue which is called subendocardial layer.

3) The myocardium is thick and forms by a large amount of cardiac muscle fibers.

4) The epicardium is composed of a single layer of mesothelial cells and a thin layer of loose connective tissue containing both elastic and collagenous fibers. Fibroblasts, fat cells and blood vessels are also present in the epicardium.

(2) High power：

The Purkinje fibers are much larger than the usual cardiac muscle fibers in the myocardium. The sarcoplasm is stained paler due to the paucity of myofibrils. The nuclei of the fibers are centrally located.

B. Identification requirements

(1) Layers of endocardium.

(2) Myocardium.

(3) Epicardium.

(4) Purkinje fibers.

cardiac
valve

6. Cardiac valve

A. Staining　HE.

（1）Low power：The surface of the cardiac valve is lined by endothelium，under which dense connective tissues can be found.

（2）High power：

1）The dense connective tissue contains purple-stained collagenous fibers and dark nuclei of fibroblasts.

2）A few smooth muscle fibers can be observed beneath the endothelium at the root of the cardiac valve.

B. Identification requirements

（1）Cardiac valve.

（2）Ventricular.

（3）Atrial surfaces.

Part II　Questions for Review

（1）Briefly describe the composition of the circulatory system.

（2）Briefly describe the structural features of different types of arteries and veins.

（3）Briefly describe the classification of the capillaries；what are the differences among the three types of capillaries.

（4）Briefly describe the structural components of the heart wall and the components，distribution，and structural features of the conducting system.

Part III　Pictures Questions for Review

Fig.8 - 1　　　　Fig.8 - 2　　　　Fig.8 - 3　　　　Fig.8 - 4

（Li Dongmei，Han Xiaodong，Ding Weidong）

第九章

免 疫 系 统

学习要点

☞ 淋巴细胞的主要类型、单核吞噬细胞系统的概念。

☞ 弥散淋巴组织与淋巴小结的结构。

☞ 胸腺的结构和功能。

☞ 淋巴结的结构和功能。

☞ 脾的结构和功能。

一、实 验 内 容

淋巴结

（一）淋巴结

1. 染色　　HE。

（1）低倍镜：

1）表面由薄层结缔组织构成的被膜；其中可见输入淋巴管,结缔组织伸入实质构成小梁。淋巴结实质由周边深染的皮质和中央浅染的髓质构成。

2）皮质位于被膜下方,皮质浅层有染色较深的淋巴小结,淋巴小结之间有少量弥散淋巴组织。

3）皮质深层为副皮质区,由深染的弥散淋巴组织构成,可见毛细血管后微静脉。

4）浅层淋巴小结与被膜、小梁之间有浅染的疏松裂隙为皮质淋巴窦,包括被膜下窦和小梁周窦。

5）髓质由髓索和髓窦构成,髓索由深染的索条状淋巴组织构成,有分支交织成网;髓窦是位于髓索之间的淋巴窦。

（2）高倍镜：

1）淋巴窦窦壁由单层扁平细胞构成;窦腔内有网状细胞、淋巴细胞和巨噬细胞。

2）淋巴细胞核大而圆,深染,胞质少,强嗜碱性。

3）巨噬细胞形态不规则,胞质深染,胞质内可见吞噬颗粒。

4）网状细胞有突起,胞质着色浅,核椭圆形居中,核仁明显。

2. 要求识别

（1）被膜、小梁。

（2）皮质、髓质。

（3）淋巴小结、副皮质区。

（4）髓索、髓窦。

（5）毛细血管后微静脉。

（6）淋巴细胞、巨噬细胞、网状细胞。

（二）脾

脾

1.染色　　HE。

（1）低倍镜：

1）脾脏表面有被膜，并由间皮覆盖，间皮下方结缔组织较厚，内含平滑肌纤维，结缔组织伸入实质形成小梁，呈块状或条索状分散在实质内，内含小梁动、静脉。

2）白髓散在于实质中，呈紫蓝色团块状，由脾小体和动脉周围淋巴鞘构成；动脉周围淋巴鞘由T细胞围绕中央动脉构成，动脉周围淋巴鞘一侧可见到脾小体，主要由B细胞组成。

3）红髓位于白髓之间，呈红色，其中有许多不规则裂隙，即脾血窦，脾血窦之间细胞较密集的部分为脾索，由富含血细胞的淋巴组织所构成。

（2）高倍镜：动脉周围淋巴鞘中可见1～2个血管腔，腔小壁厚，中膜由环形排列的平滑肌构成，为中央动脉。

2.要求识别

（1）被膜、小梁。

（2）动脉周围淋巴鞘、中央动脉。

（3）脾小体、脾索、脾血窦。

（三）胸腺

胸腺

1.染色　　HE。

（1）低倍镜：

1）胸腺表面有结缔组织被膜，结缔组织伸入实质形成小叶间隔，将实质分成许多不完全分离的胸腺小叶。

2）胸腺小叶周边由深染的皮质构成，中间为浅染的髓质。

3）小叶髓质中有大小不等的浅红色胸腺小体。

（2）高倍镜：

1）皮质由密集的胸腺细胞和少量的胸腺上皮细胞构成，可见巨噬细胞。胸腺细胞体积小，核圆，深染，胞质不易分辨。

2）胸腺上皮细胞核大，椭圆形，着色浅，胞质浅染。

3）胸腺小体大小不一，由多层扁平的胸腺上皮细胞呈同心圆围成，大多数细胞开始退化，细胞核固缩，小体中心的细胞完全退化和死亡，呈粉红色均质状。

2.要求识别

（1）被膜、小叶间隔。

（2）皮质、髓质。

（3）胸腺小体。

（4）胸腺上皮细胞。

扁桃体

（四）扁桃体

1. 染色　　HE。

低倍镜：

1）上皮为未角化的复层扁平上皮；上皮内有淋巴细胞浸润。

2）上皮下固有层内和隐窝周围有淋巴组织；其中淋巴小结内可见生发中心，小结之间是弥散淋巴组织。

3）被膜结缔组织伸入淋巴组织形成小梁。

4）被膜外可见淡蓝色黏液性腺泡。

2. 要求识别

（1）上皮。

（2）淋巴组织。

（3）隐窝。

（4）被膜。

二、复习思考题

（1）简述淋巴细胞的分类和淋巴细胞再循环的概念。

（2）简述淋巴结的结构和功能。

（3）简述胸腺的结构和功能。

（4）简述脾脏的结构和功能。

（5）简述血-胸腺屏障的组成和功能。

三、图片思考题

图 9-1　　　　　　　　图 9-2

（李冬梅　韩晓冬　丁卫东）

Chapter 9

IMMUNE SYSTEM

Learning Points

☞ The major kinds of lymphocytes, the concept of the mononuclear phagocyte system.

☞ The structure of diffuse lymphoid tissue and lymphoid nodules.

☞ The structure of the thymus and its function.

☞ The structure of the lymph node and its function.

☞ The structure of the spleen and its function.

Part I   Experiment Contents

lymph node

1. Lymph node

A. Staining   HE.

(1) Low power:

1) The lymph node is surrounded by a capsule of connective tissue, from which the connective tissue extends into the interior to form trabeculae. The afferent lymphatic vessels are located in the capsule; it is composed of two main parts: the palely stained peripheral cortex and the deeply stained central medulla.

2) The cortex is located beneath the capsule, which consists of deeply stained lymph nodules and palely stained diffuse lymphoid tissue between the adjacent lymph nodules.

3) The inner, deep cortex is known as the paracortex which consists of the diffuse lymphoid tissue; postcapillary venules can be identified there.

4) Nodules are separated from the capsule and trabeculae by channel-like spaces, i.e. lymph sinuses which are divided into subcapsular and peritrabecular sinuses.

5) The medulla consists of medullary cords and medullary sinuses. The medullary cords are the deeply stained strands of densely aggregated lymphoid tissues which branch and connect each other. The relatively cell-free areas between the medullary cords are medullary sinuses.

(2) High power:

1) Lymph sinuses are lined with simple squamous epithelium; the lumen contains lymphocytes, reticular cells and macrophages.

2) Lymphocytes are hyperbasophilic cells with deeply stained, scanty cytoplasm and large, round nuclei.

3) Macrophages are irregular in shape with deeply stained cytoplasm containing engulfed granular particles.

4) Reticular cells have processes with pink-stained cytoplasm. They have centrally placed round or ovoid nuclei and prominent nucleoli.

B. Identification requirements

(1) Capsule and trabeculae.

(2) Cortex and medulla.

(3) Lymph nodules and paracortex.

(4) The medullary cords and medullary sinuses.

(5) Postcapillary venules.

(6) Lymphocytes, macrophages and reticular cells.

2. Spleen

spleen

A. Staining   HE.

(1) Low power:

1) The surface of the spleen is covered by a capsule which consists of the mesothelium and the dense connective tissue which is relatively thick and contains a few smooth muscle cells in addition to fibrous elements. It extends into parenchyma and forms trabeculae, which further branches and anastomoses to form a three-dimensional supporting network which contains blood vessels.

2) The white pulp scatters throughout the spleen and contains round or ellipsoid bodies that are deeply stained blue. They are composed of splenic nodules and the periarterial lymphatic sheath. The periarterial lymphatic sheath contains dense lymphatic tissue cords around the central artery, next to which are the splenic nodules which are composed of B lymphocytes.

3) The red pulp lies between the white pulp and contains splenic cords and sinusoids. Splenic cords lie around the sinusoids and are composed of lymphatic tissue with numerous blood cells. Sinusoids are large irregular lumens containing RBC.

(2) High power: 1 to 2 lumens of blood vessels may be seen in the periarterial lymphatic sheath. The lumen is small with a thick wall. They are central arteries.

B. Identification requirements

(1) Capsule and trabeculae.

(2) Periarterial lymphatic sheath and the central artery.

(3) Splenic nodules, splenic cords and sinusoids.

3. Thymus

thymus

A. Staining　　HE.

（1）Low power：

1）The thymus is surrounded by a thin connective tissue capsule，from which trabeculae extend into parenchyma and separate it into numerous incomplete lobules of various sizes and shapes.

2）The periphery of each lobule stains deeply and is called cortex，while the inner，central portion stains pale，called medulla.

3）In the central region of the medulla，there are a number of red-stained thymic corpuscles.

（2）High power：

1）Cortex is mainly composed of a large number of closely aggregated lymphocytes，a few thymic epithelial cells and macrophages. Lymphocytes are small with round，dark blue nuclei and scanty cytoplasm.

2）Thymic epithelial cells contain large pale nuclei and pale-stained cytoplasm.

3）The thymic corpuscle is a small round corpuscle of various sizes，and each lobule contains one or more corpuscles in number. The corpuscle is composed of flattened epithelial reticular cells arranged concentrically，most of which degenerate with shrunk nuclei. The cells at the corpuscle center completely degenerate and die presenting a red homogenous structure.

B. Identification requirements

（1）Capsule and interlobular septa.

（2）Cortex and medulla.

（3）Thymic corpuscle.

（4）Thymic epithelial cell.

4. Palatine tonsil

palatine tonsil

A. Staining　　HE.

Low power：

1）The epithelium over the tonsil is made up of non-keratinized stratified squamous epithelium，which is infiltrated by lymphocytes and may infold in some places to form crypts.

2）The deeply stained blue portion underlying the epithelium is lymphoid tissue，out of which is the pink-stained capsule. The lymphatic tissue is distributed in the lamina propria beneath the epithelium and around the crypts. It forms many lymphatic nodules arranged in rows and surrounded by diffuse lymphatic tissue.

3）Capsule is made up of loose connective tissue at the outside of the lymphatic tissue. Sometimes the connective tissue extends into the tonsil to form trabeculae.

4）A few blue mucous glands may be seen outside the capsule.

B. Identification requirements

（1）Epithelium.

（2）Lymphatic tissue.

（3）Crypts.

（4）Capsule.

Part II　Questions for Review

（1）Briefly describe the classification of lymphocytes and the significance of lymphocyte recirculation.

（2）Briefly describe the structure of the lymph node and its function.

（3）Briefly describe the structure of the thymus and its function.

（4）Briefly describe the structure of the spleen and its function.

（5）Briefly describe the structure and function of the blood-thymus barrier.

Part III　Pictures Questions for Review

Fig.9 - 1　　　　Fig.9 - 2

（Li Dongmei，Han Xiaodong，Ding Weidong）

第十章

皮　肤

学习要点

☞ 皮肤的组织结构与功能。

☞ 表皮的分层与角化过程。

☞ 黑素细胞、朗格汉斯细胞的分布、结构和功能。

☞ 真皮的组织结构。

☞ 各种皮肤附属器的结构特点与功能。

一、实验内容

厚皮肤

（一）厚皮肤

1. 染色　　HE。

（1）低倍镜：

1）皮肤由浅至深分3层：表皮、真皮和皮下组织。

2）表皮为角化的复层扁平上皮，没有血管，由表面向深层又可分为：角质层、透明层、颗粒层、棘层和基底层。

3）真皮位于表皮下面，由富含血管的致密结缔组织构成，可分为乳头层和网织层。

4）真皮的结缔组织嵌入表皮基部形成乳头，此层纤维较细，排列致密，内含丰富的毛细血管或触觉小体。

5）网织层位于真皮深层，较厚，有纵横交错的胶原纤维束，与乳头层没有明显界限，此层含较大的血管、神经、汗腺的导管和分泌部。

6）在真皮和皮下组织交界处还可见环层小体，呈卵圆形或圆形，中央有一均质状的棒状或圆形结构，周围有多层同心圆排列的扁平细胞。

（2）高倍镜：

1）角质层位于表皮最浅层，为多层已完全角化的扁平细胞，细胞核消失，胞质中充满嗜酸性角蛋白，染成深红色，细胞界限不清。

2）透明层由2～3层扁平细胞组成，细胞呈均质状，染成浅红色，核已退化消失。

3）颗粒层由2～3层棱形细胞构成，胞质内有深蓝色嗜碱性透明角质颗粒，与透明层之间有裂隙。

4）棘层由4～10层多边形细胞组成，核呈圆形或卵圆形，染色较浅，相邻细胞有棘。

5）基底层位于表皮最底层,为单层立方或矮柱状细胞,胞质染成紫蓝色。

6）真皮乳头层中有卵圆形的触觉小体,小体外包薄层结缔组织被囊,内有数个横行排列的扁平细胞;有髓神经纤维的分支进入小体,在扁平细胞之间盘旋上行。

7）真皮深层和皮下组织可见成群的汗腺导管断面和分泌部;导管的管腔较小,管壁由 2～3 层矮柱状细胞围成,染色较深;分泌部管腔较大,由立方形细胞构成。

2．要求识别

(1) 角质层、透明层、颗粒层、棘层、基底层。

(2) 乳头层、网织层。

(3) 触觉小体、环层小体。

(4) 汗腺的分泌部和导管。

（二）薄皮肤

薄皮肤

1．染色　　HE。

低倍镜:

1）层次结构与厚皮肤相似,但表皮较薄。

2）角质层较薄,透明层、颗粒层不明显,棘层薄。

3）真皮较厚,在真皮内可见许多毛囊、立毛肌、皮脂腺和汗腺。

4）毛囊分上皮根鞘和结缔组织鞘,中间被染成棕黄色的部分为毛根,有的切面已脱落,为一空腔。

5）毛囊的一侧可见一束平滑肌,为立毛肌;立毛肌与毛囊之间接近基底部可见皮脂腺。

2．要求识别

(1) 毛囊,毛根。

(2) 上皮根鞘、结缔组织鞘。

(3) 立毛肌。

(4) 皮脂腺。

二、复习思考题

(1) 简述表皮的分层。

(2) 皮肤的附属结构有哪些?

(3) 简述触觉小体和环层小体的结构和功能。

三、图片思考题

图 10-1

图 10-2

（李冬梅　韩晓冬　丁卫东）

Chapter 10

SKIN

Learning Points

☞ The Structure and function of skin.

☞ The layers and keratinization of epidermis.

☞ The distribution, structure and function of the Langerhans cells and melanocytes.

☞ The structure of dermis.

☞ The Structural characteristics and related functions of skin appendages.

Part I   Experiment Contents

1. Thick skin

A. Staining   HE.

(1) Low power:

thick skin

1) The skin is divided into three layers from the free surface to the base: epidermis, dermis and hypodermis.

2) The epidermis is stratified squamous keratinized epithelium without blood vessels and from the free surface inward consists of five layers: stratum corneum, stratum lucidum, stratum granulosum, stratum spinosum, and stratum basale.

3) The dermis is composed of dense connective tissue beneath the epidermis. It can be subdivided into the papillary layer and reticular layer.

4) The papillary layer is the connective tissue that projects into the epidermis. This layer consists mainly of fine collagenous fibers, reticular fibers and elastic fibers. Some papillae may contain special sensory terminals, Meissner's corpuscle; some contain blood vessels.

5) The reticular layer consists mainly of bundles of coarse collagenous fibers running in various directions. It also contains larger blood vessels, nerves, ducts and the secretory portions of the sweat glands.

6) Lamellar corpuscles are located deeply in the dermis and in the subcutaneous tissue. They are round or elliptical and composed of a number of concentric lamellae of flattened cells. A thin layer of dense connective tissue encloses the lamellar corpuscle.

In the center of the corpuscle is an inner bulb.

(2) High power:

1) The stratum corneum is composed of a number of layers of flattened, dead cells, the nuclei of which are no longer visible. The cytoplasm is packed with keratin, which is stained dark red with indistinct cell borders.

2) The stratum lucidum is a pale layer that is stained pink, and the nuclei of the cells in this layer have disappeared.

3) The stratum granulosum is formed by 2 to 3 layers of flattened cells filled with keratohyalin granules stained deeply with blue-black and hematoxylin.

4) The stratum spinosum has 4 to 10 layers of polyhedral cells. The cells there have fine intercellular clefts separating the cells from one another.

5) The stratum basale is a single layer of cuboidal cells, forming the deepest layer of the epithelium. The cytoplasm is stained purple blue.

6) Tactile corpuscles (Meissner's Corpuscles) are oval and surrounded by a capsular layer of connective tissue, and consist of a spiral non-myelinated branch of large myelinated sensory fibers. The cells forming the encapsulated layers seem to be largely horizontally situated, and the nerve fibers wind upwards between these encapsulated cells.

7) The ducts of sweat gland are composed of two layers of cuboidal cells, which are more darkly stained, and these cells are smaller so that the nuclei are more closely packed. The secretory portion of the gland is thicker in diameter than the duct and lined by a simple short columnar or cuboidal epithelium.

B. Identification Requirements

(1) Stratum corneum, stratum lucidum, stratum granulosum, stratum spinosum, and stratum basale.

(2) Papillary layer and reticular layer.

(3) Meissner's corpuscle, Lamellar corpuscle.

(4) The secretory portion and the duct of eccrine sweat gland.

2. Thin skin

thin skin

A. Staining   HE.

Low power:

1) The structure of the thin skin is similar to that of the thick skin, but the epidermis is distinctively thinner.

2) The stratum lucidum and the stratum granulosum of the thin skin are often less well developed, the stratum corneum may be quite thin, and the stratum spinosum is thinner.

3) The dermis is thicker and contains hair follicles, arrector pili muscle, sebaceous glands and sweat glands.

4）Each hair consists of a hair shaft which projects above the surface of the epidermis and a root which is stained brownish-yellow and embedded in a hair follicle. The hair follicle is made up of epithelium and connective tissue.

5）Arrector pili muscles are bundles of smooth muscle cells. The sebaceous glands are located between an arrector pili muscle and its hair follicle.

B. Identification requirements

（1）Hair shaft and hair root.

（2）Epithelial sheath and connective tissue sheath.

（3）Arrector pili muscle.

（4）Sebaceous gland.

Part II   Question for Review

（1）Briefly describe the layers of epidermis.

（2）What are the structures of the skin appendages?

（3）Briefly describe the structure and function of the tactile corpuscle and the lamellar corpuscle.

Part III   Pictures Questions for Review

Fig.10 - 1   Fig.10 - 2

（Li Dongmei，Han Xiaodong，Ding Weidong）

第十一章

消　化　管

学习要点

☞ 消化管的一般结构。

☞ 舌乳头的结构和类型,味蕾的分布、结构和功能,牙的结构。

☞ 食管的结构特点。

☞ 胃的结构,胃底腺的结构和功能,胃黏膜的自我保护机制。

☞ 小肠的结构,小肠各段结构特点,结肠、阑尾和直肠的结构特点。

一、实 验 内 容

食管

(一) 食管(横切面)

1. 染色　　HE。

(1) 低倍镜:从黏膜上皮向外膜方向依次观察各层结构。

1) 黏膜层:与黏膜下层一起向管腔内突起形成皱襞。其中上皮为未角化的复层扁平上皮,较厚,基底部起伏不平。固有层为薄层细密的结缔组织,并突入上皮深面形成许多乳头,其中含有丰富的小血管和食管腺导管,部分切片中可见淋巴组织以及食管贲门腺。黏膜肌由一层纵行平滑肌构成,较发达,随黏膜皱襞起伏。

2) 黏膜下层:由疏松结缔组织构成,染色浅淡,内含丰富的血管、食管腺的腺泡及导管、黏膜下神经丛等。

3) 肌层:分内环、外纵两层肌肉,肌纤维类型因取材部位,即上、中、下三段不同而异,试判断标本取自食管的哪一段。

4) 外膜:为纤维膜。

(2) 高倍镜:

1) 仔细观察黏膜下层的食管腺,腺泡为黏液性。

2) 区分小动脉和食管腺导管的切面。

3) 观察肌层中肌纤维的类型。

2. 要求识别

(1) 食管壁的分层。

（2）各层的结构特点。

（3）食管腺和导管。

胃

（二）胃

1. 染色　　HE。

（1）低倍镜：从黏膜向浆膜方向依次观察。

1）黏膜层：其中上皮为单层柱状上皮,细胞境界清楚,细胞顶部色浅透明,因其黏原颗粒在制片过程中呈空泡状。核卵圆形,位于基底部。上皮凹陷形成较浅而阔的胃小凹,在黏膜浅层可见胃小凹的各种切面。固有层内有大量的胃底腺,因切面的不同,腺体被切成各种断面,制片时组织收缩,故腺腔不明显。腺体之间有少量的结缔组织、淋巴组织和散在的平滑肌纤维。选择一个典型的纵切面的胃底腺,区分出腺体的颈部、体部和底部。黏膜肌层较薄,由内环、外纵两层平滑肌构成。

2）黏膜下层为疏松结缔组织,可见血管、神经和黏膜下神经丛等结构。

3）肌层较厚,由内斜、中环、外纵三层平滑肌构成。中环、外纵肌层间可见肌间神经丛。

4）外膜为浆膜,由薄层结缔组织和间皮构成。

（2）高倍镜：着重观察胃底腺的腺体细胞。

1）主细胞：主要分布在腺体的体部或底部。细胞呈柱状,核圆形,位于细胞基底部,胞质嗜碱性,染成浅蓝色。

2）壁细胞：主要分布在腺体的颈部或体部。细胞较大,呈圆形或锥体形,细胞核圆形,位于细胞中央,胞质嗜酸性,染成鲜红色。

3）颈黏液细胞：分布在腺体的颈部,数量较少,呈柱形或烧瓶形,胞质染色浅,核扁圆形位于基底部,由于该细胞量少,在切片上不容易分辨。

2. 要求识别

（1）胃壁的分层及各层的结构。

（2）胃皱襞。

（3）胃小凹。

（4）胃腺的主细胞和壁细胞。

（5）观察神经丛,区分神经纤维的横断面和血管的横断面。

十二指肠

（三）十二指肠

1. 染色　　HE。

（1）低倍镜：从腔面的黏膜层向浆膜层逐层观察。

1）黏膜层：其中上皮为单层柱状,主要的细胞为吸收细胞,其表面有纹状缘,核椭圆形,位于细胞基底部。杯状细胞夹杂在吸收细胞之间,呈高脚酒杯状,上皮与固有层向腔内突起形成绒毛,上皮向固有层凹陷形成肠腺。由于绒毛在肠腔内长短不一,走向不同,切片中可见到各种不同切面,可根据中心的结缔组织来辨认。绒毛中的固有层为疏松结缔组织,内含丰富的肠腺、毛细血管、分散的平滑肌、淋巴细胞、浆细胞和巨噬细胞等。固有层内有许多不同切面的肠腺,而结缔组织较少。有时可见孤立淋巴小结。黏膜肌为内环、外纵排列的平滑肌,较薄。

2) 黏膜下层：为疏松结缔组织，含有较大的血管、神经、十二指肠腺等。十二指肠腺为盘曲成团的管状腺，腺导管穿过黏膜肌通入肠腺的底部。试比较十二指肠腺与肠腺在结构和位置上的不同。

3) 肌层：内环、外纵两层平滑肌，外纵肌较薄，肌层之间可见少量结缔组织和肌间神经丛。

4) 浆膜：由薄层结缔组织和间皮构成，但十二指肠附着于后腹壁处是纤维膜。

（2）高倍镜：

1) 上皮游离面的纹状缘，呈带状，红色发亮。可见吸收细胞和杯状细胞，内分泌细胞显示不出来，杯状细胞较少，呈高脚酒杯状，散在于吸收细胞之间，核呈三角形，位于基底部。

2) 绒毛的结构：中轴为固有层的结缔组织，内含中央乳糜管、毛细血管、淋巴细胞、浆细胞和分散的平滑肌等，平滑肌的长轴与绒毛的长轴一致，中央乳糜管因壁薄而容易塌陷，故不易识别。

3) 肠腺主要由吸收细胞、杯状细胞和少数帕内特细胞构成。

2. 要求识别

（1）十二指肠各层的结构特点。

（2）肠绒毛。

（3）肠腺和肠绒毛在切片上的不同。

直肠

（四）直肠

1. 染色　　HE。

低倍镜：从肠腔的黏膜层向浆膜层逐层观察。

1) 黏膜层：其中上皮为单层柱状上皮，夹有大量的杯状细胞。固有层充满大肠腺，腺细胞以杯状细胞为主，夹有柱状细胞。淋巴小结分散存在，有的淋巴小结可突破黏膜肌，伸入黏膜下层。黏膜肌层：内环、外纵两层平滑肌，皱襞顶部的黏膜肌较厚。

2) 黏膜下层：疏松结缔组织，含血管、神经和脂肪细胞等，可见孤立淋巴小结和黏膜下神经丛。

3) 肌层：内环、外纵两层平滑肌，外纵肌层较厚，肌层间可见肌间神经丛。

4) 浆膜：直肠上部的前面和侧面为浆膜，其余部分为纤维膜。

2. 要求识别

（1）直肠壁的分层及各层结构。

（2）大肠腺。

二、复 习 思 考 题

（1）简述消化管的一般结构。

（2）黏膜下层有腺体的器官有哪些？

（3）简述食管、胃、小肠的结构特点及功能。

（4）小肠内扩大吸收面积的结构有哪些？

三、图片思考题

图 11-1

图 11-2

图 11-3

图 11-4

（魏剑锋）

Chapter 11

DIGESTIVE TRACT

Learning Points

☞ The general structure of digestive tract.

☞ The structure and types of tongue papillae, the distribution, structure and function of the taste buds, and the structure of the teeth.

☞ The structural characteristics of the esophagus.

☞ The structure of the stomach, the structure and function of the gastric glands, and the mechanism of the self-protection of gastric mucosa.

☞ The structure of the small intestine, the structural features of the duodenum, jejunum and ileum, and the structural features of the colon, appendix and rectum.

Part I　Experiment Contents

1. Esophagus

esophagus

A. Staining　　HE.

(1) Low power: Observe the wall structure from the free surface of mucosa to the adventitia.

1) Mucous layers together with submucosa forms the plica.

Epithelium is nonkeratinized stratified squamous epithelium which is thick and undulating at the base.

Lamina propria is a thin layer of loose connective tissue and located beneath the epithelium rich in small blood vessels and the ducts of esophageal glands can be observed in it.

Muscularis mucosa is a layer of longitudinal smooth muscle fibers, well developed and becomes undulated with the mucosal folds.

2) Submucosa is composed of loose connective tissue, pale-stained and rich in blood vessels. The acini and ducts of esophageal glands and submucous nerve plexus can be observed.

3) Muscularis externa consists of inner circular and outer longitudinal muscles.

The type of muscle fibers varies in different parts upper，middle，lower. Try to determine from which part of the esophagus the specimen was prepared?

4）Adventitia is a fibrous membrane.

（2）High power：

1）Observe the esophageal glands of the submucosa carefully. The acini are mucous.

2）Pay attention to the distinctions between the small arteries and the esophageal gland ducts.

3）Observe the types of muscle fibers in the muscularis externa.

B. Identification requirements

（1）The layers of esophagus.

（2）The structural characteristics of each layer.

（3）Esophageal gland and its duct.

2. Stomach

stomach

A. Staining   HE.

（1）Low power：Observe the wall structures from the free surface of mocosa to serosa.

1）Mucosa：Epithelium is simple columnar，whose cells are lightly stained and even transparent. The mucous granules in the epithelial cells are vaculated during prepartion. Their nuclei are oval and located near the base. The epithelium invaginates to form the shallow and wide gastric pits. Various profiles of the gastric pits can be observed in this slide.

Lamina propria contains a large amount of gastric glands, which show different profiles in the slide. It is difficult to identify the boundary of the gastric glands due to the contraction of the tissues during the preparation of the specimen. A small amount of connective tissue，lymphatic tissue and smooth muscle intersperse between the gastric glands. Select one typical longitudinal section of gastric glands and identify its neck，body and bottom.

Muscularis mucosa is thin and consists of an inner circular and an outer longitudinal layer of smooth muscle.

2）Submucosa is formed by loose connective tissue containing blood vessels，nerves and submucosal nerve plexus.

3）Mucularis externa is thick and composed of three layers of smooth muscle. The nerve plexus is visible between the middle circular and outer longitudinal muscle layers.

4）Adventitia is a serous membrane constituted by a thin layer of connective tissue and mesothelium.

（2）High power：Pay attention to the glandular cells in the body of gastric gland.

1）The chief cells are mainly distributed in the body or bottom of the gastric glands. The cell is low columnar and the nucleus is round, located in the basal part of the cell and the basophilic cytoplasm is stained light blue.

2) Parietal cells are mainly distributed in the neck or body of the glands. They are spheroidal or cone-shaped and their nuclei are also round and located in the center. Their eosinophilic cytoplasm is stained bright red.

3) Mucous neck cells are usually distributed in the neck of glands. They are cylindrical or flask-shaped and their cytoplasm are stained pale. The nucleus is flattened round at the base of the cell, which is not easy to be observed since its number is few.

B. Identification requirements

(1) The structure of gastric layers.

(2) Gastric folds.

(3) Gastric pits.

(4) The chief cells and parietal cells of the gastric glands.

(5) Observe the nerve plexus and identify the cross-section of the nerve fibers and blood vessels.

3. Duodenum

duodenum

A. Staining   HE.

(1) Low power: Observe the wall structures from the free surface of mucosa to serosa.

1) Mucosa: Epithelium is simple columnar. The absorptive cells have striated border and ovoid nuclei located near the base. The goblet cells are irregularly scattered among the absorptive cells, which is goblet-like in shape. The epithelium and lamina propria protrude into the lumen and form the intestinal villi. The intestinal villi have varying lengths and different orientations. So a wide variety of profiles can be found in a section.

Lamina propria of the intesinal villi is similar to loose connective tissue, which contains a lot of intestinal glands, blood vessels, scattered smooth muscle, lymphocytes, plasma cells and macrophages, etc. The glands have many different profiles in the lamina propria. Sometimes the isolated lymphoid nodules are visible here.

Muscularis mucosa is thinner and composed of inner circular and outer longitudinal layers of smooth muscles.

2) Submucosa is a loose connective tissue containing larger blood vessels, nerves and duodenal glands. Duodenal gland is a group of coiled tubular gland, and the gland duct penetrates the muscularis mucosa into the bottom of the intestinal glands. Try to compare the differences between duodenal glands and intestine glands.

3) Muscularis externa is composed of two layers, namely the inner circular and

outer longitudinal smooth muscle. The outer longitudinal muscle layer is thinner and a small amount of connective tissue and the myenteric nerve plexus are visible between the two layers of smooth muscle.

4) Adventitia is constituted by a thin layer of connective tissue covered by mesothelium, while the part of duodenum attached to the posterior abdominal wall is a fibrous membrane.

(2) High power:

1) The striated border of the epithelial cells looks like pink shiny ribbon. Absorptive cells and goblet cells are visible, while the endocrine cells are not. Goblet cells are fewer than absorptive cells. A few goblet cells scatter among the absorptive cells, The basal part of the goblet cell has a triangular or crescent nucleus.

2) The structure of the cores of the intestinal villi is the connective tissue of the lamina propria, including central lacteal, capillaries, lymphocytes, plasma cells and the dispersed smooth muscle fibers etc. The central lacteal wall is thin and easy to collapse, so it is difficult to be observed.

3) The intestinal glands are composed of mainly absorptive cells, goblet cells and a few Paneth cells.

B. Identification requirements

(1) The structural features of the four principal layers of the duodenum.

(2) Intestinal villus.

(3) The differences between intestinal glands and intestinal villi in section.

4. Rectum

rectum

A. Staining   HE.

Low power: Observe the wall structure from the free surface of mucosa to serosa.

1) Mucosa: Epithelium is a simple columnar epithelium and a large number of goblet cells scatter among them.

Lamina propria is full of intestinal gland. The majority of the cells in the gland are goblet cells while the minority is absorptive cells. The lymphoid nodules exist dispersively, and some lymphoid nodules break through muscularis mucosa and stretch to the submucosa.

Muscularis mucosa contains the inner circular and outer longitudinal layers of smooth muscle.

2) Submucosa is a kind of loose connective tissue, which contains blood vessels, nerves and fat cells, etc. Isolated lymphoid nodules and submucosal nerve plexus are visible here.

3) Muscularis externa has two layers, namely the inner circular and outer thick longitudinal smooth muscle, and the myenteric nerve plexus between the two layers is

possible to be distinguished.

4) Serosa is located in the ventral and lateral aspects of the upper rectum. The remaining portion is covered by fibrous membrane.

B. Identification requirements

(1) The structure of rectum wall and its four principal layers.

(2) Intestinal gland of the rectum.

Part II   Question for Review

(1) Briefly describe the general structures of the digestive tract.

(2) What are the organs that have glands in their submucosa?

(3) Briefly describe the structural features and functions of the esophagus, stomach and small intestine.

(4) What are the special structures that expand the surface area of small intestine?

Part III   Pictures Questions for Review

Fig.11 - 1   Fig.11 - 2   Fig.11 - 3   Fig.11 - 4

(Wei Jianfeng)

第十二章

消 化 腺

学习要点

☞ 胰的形态结构和功能。
☞ 肝的形态结构和功能。
☞ 肝细胞的形态结构和功能。

一、实 验 内 容

胰腺

（一）胰腺

1. 染色　　HE。

（1）低倍镜：

　　1）胰腺表面有结缔组织,但不形成明显被膜,结缔组织深入实质将胰腺分隔成大小不等的小叶。

　2）小叶内有大量染成紫红色的浆液性腺泡。

　3）导管和腺泡之间散在的大小不等的浅色细胞团即为胰岛。

（2）高倍镜：

　　1）腺泡属于浆液性腺泡,腺细胞呈锥体形,核圆形位于基底部,基部胞质呈嗜碱性,细胞顶部含嗜酸性颗粒,染成红色。腺泡中央有泡心细胞,细胞较小,胞质染色较淡,细胞界限不清,可见圆形或卵圆形的细胞核,色浅,位于细胞中央。有时可见泡心细胞与闰管相连。

　　2）小叶内可见由单层扁平或单层立方上皮构成的闰管,以及由单层立方上皮构成的小叶内导管,无纹状管,小叶间结缔组织内可见小叶间导管和主导管（只有一条主导管）,管壁由单层柱状上皮构成,中间夹有杯状细胞。

　　3）胰岛细胞排列成大小不等且形状不规则的团索,染色浅,分散在腺泡之间。构成胰岛的三种细胞不能区分,在细胞团索间可见丰富的毛细血管。

2. 要求识别

（1）浆液性腺泡。

（2）泡心细胞。

（3）各级导管。

（4）胰岛。

肝

（二）肝

1.染色　　HE。

（1）低倍镜：

1）表面为致密结缔组织的被膜，大部分被膜的表面可见间皮。人肝的肝小叶间结缔组织很少，故小叶的分界不明显，相邻肝小叶的肝索似乎彼此相连。

2）观察肝小叶时，应先找到中央静脉，其位于小叶中央，管壁不完整，管腔近似圆形，衬有内皮，腔中常有血细胞。肝索以中央静脉为中心向四周呈放射状排列，肝索的分支互相吻合成网，不规则的网眼间隙为肝血窦，彼此呈网状沟通，至小叶中央汇入中央静脉。

3）门管区位于几个肝小叶相邻间的结缔组织内，可同时见到三种伴行的管道：小叶间动脉、小叶间静脉和小叶间胆管。

（2）高倍镜：

1）中央静脉位于小叶中央，管腔比较规则，管壁薄，因有血窦的开口而不完整，可见扁平的内皮细胞核。

2）肝索由肝细胞排列而成，细胞呈多边形，体积较大，界限清楚，核圆形位于中央，染色浅，有1～2个核仁，肝索中常见有双核细胞和核大的多倍体细胞。

3）肝血窦窦壁为单层扁平上皮，上皮细胞核扁圆，染色深，并略突向窦腔，胞质很少，呈粉红色条状贴近肝索。窦腔内可见库普弗细胞（Kupffer cell，又称肝巨噬细胞），其星形突起与窦壁的内皮细胞相连，核大呈椭圆形或不规则形，胞质丰富，染成红色。窦腔中还可见各种血细胞。

4）认真鉴别门管区三种伴行管道的横断面。小叶间胆管：管径较细，由单层立方或单层柱状上皮围成，核圆居中，染色较深；小叶间动脉：管径细，壁厚，内皮外可见数层环行平滑肌；小叶间静脉：管径最粗，腔大壁薄，腔形不规则，管壁由内皮、薄层结缔组织及散在的平滑肌构成。

2.要求识别

（1）肝被膜。

（2）肝小叶的结构（中央静脉、肝索、肝血窦、肝巨噬细胞）。

（3）门管区的位置和结构（小叶间胆管、小叶间动脉、小叶间静脉）。

二、复习思考题

（1）腮腺与胰腺外分泌部有哪些区别？

（2）简述肝小叶的组成。

（3）肝门管区有哪三种管道的断面？

三、图片思考题

图 12 - 1

图 12 - 2

（孙　申）

Chapter 12

DIGESTIVE GLAND

Learning Points

☞ The structure and function of the pancreas.
☞ The structure and function of the liver.
☞ The structure and function of the liver cells.

Part I   Experiment Contents

pancreas

1. Pancreas

A. Staining   HE.

(1) Low power:

1) The pancreas is covered by a thin layer of connective tissue which dose not form a definite capsule and there are septa between pancreatic lobules.

2) Large amount of deep purple serous acini are located in the lobules.

3) Light-colored cell clusters of varying sizes scattered between the ducts and the acini are called Langerhans islet.

(2) High power:

1) Acinus belongs to the serous type and the gland cells are cone-shaped, the nuclei of which are round and located at the base. Their cytoplasm was basophilic at the basal area and eosinophilic at the apical part. The centroacinar cells lay in the centre of the acini and are lightly stained. Sometimes we can observe that centroacinar cells are connected with the intercalated duct.

2) Intercalated duct is formed by simple squamous epithelium or simple cuboidal epithelium. The lobular duct is composed of simple cuboidal epithelium. While there are no striated ducts, interlobular ducts and main ducts are visible in interlobular connective tissue. The wall of the main duct is formed by simple columnar epithelium interspersed with some goblet cells.

3) The round clusters or cords of the endocrine cells in the Langerhans islets are lightly stained, different in size and irregular in shape, which disperse in the exocrine

portion. The three types of cells in the islet cannot be distinguished and capillaries are prominent in the islet.

B. Identification requirements

(1) The structure of the Langerhans islets.

(2) Serous acini.

(3) Centroacinar cells.

(4) Ducts.

liver

2. Liver

A. Staining　　HE.

(1) Low power：

1) The surface of the liver is covered by dense connective tissue and mesothelium. Since very little connective tissue exists between the hepatic lobule, lobular boundaries are not obvious in the human liver. Hepatic cords in adjacent lobules seem to be connected with each other.

2) When observing the hepatic lobule, central vein should be found firstly. The central vein is located in the center of hepatic lobule, its wall is incomplete, its lumen is nearly circular its surface is lined with endothelium. Hepatic cord is radially arranged around the central vein and anastomoses with each other to form a network. The irregular mesh gaps are called hepatic sinusoids, which connect with each other and with the central vein.

3) Portal area is located between several adjacent hepatic lobules. In this area, three accompanying vessels, i. e. interlobular arteries, interlobular veins and interlobular bile duct can be found.

(2) High power：

1) The central vein is located in the center of the hepatic lobule. The lumen is relatively regular and the wall is thin. The endothelial nuclei are flat. The wall of the central vein is incomplete because the sinusoids open on it.

2) Hepatic cord is formed by the relatively regular arrangements of hepatocytes. The hepatocytes are polygonal and large with clear boundaries. The round nuclei are located in the center and stained light, each of which contains for 1 to 2 nucleoli. Commonly, the bi-nucleated cells and polyploid cells can be seen in the hepatic cord.

3) The wall of the hepatic sinusoids is formed by a single layer squamous cell, whose nuclei are oblate and deeply stained. What is more, the cells are slightly protruding into the sinus and contain a small amount of pink stained cytoplasm. The Kupffer cells can be observed in the sinus, their star-shaped projections connect with the endothelial cells of the sinus wall, and their nuclei are oval or irregular. Various blood cells are also visible in the sinuses.

4) Identify the cross-section of the three accompanying pipelines can be found in

portal areas. Interlobular bile ducts are composed of simple cuboidal epithelium. The nucleus is round, centrical and deeply stained. Interlobular arteries are thin in diameter and have thick wall. Several layers of circular smooth muscle are visible outside the endothelium of the interlobular arteries. Interlobular vein has irregular lumen. Its cavity is large and its wall is thin.

B. Identification requirements

(1) Liver capsule.

(2) The structure of hepatic lobule (central vein, hepatic cord, liver sinusoid and Kupffer cell).

(3) The position and structure of the portal area (interlobular bile ducts, interlobular arteries and interlobular veins).

Part II   Questions for Review

(1) What are the differences between the parotid and exocrine pancreas?

(2) Briefly describe the compositions of the hepatic lobule.

(3) What are the three ducts in hepatic portal area?

Part III   Pictures Questions for Review

Fig.12 - 1

Fig.12 - 2

(Sun shen)

第十三章

呼 吸 系 统

学习要点

☞ 肺导气部的形态、结构与功能。
☞ 肺呼吸部的形态、结构与功能。

一、实 验 内 容

（一）气管

气管

1. 染色　　HE。

（1）低倍镜：

1）黏膜上皮是假复层纤毛柱状上皮，位于基膜上。基膜下方是细密的结缔组织构成的固有层，内含弹性纤维、腺体导管、血管、淋巴组织和浆细胞等。

2）黏膜下层为疏松结缔组织，与固有层无明显界限，其中含一些混合腺及小血管。

3）外膜主要由透明软骨和结缔组织构成，其中可见 C 形的透明软骨环。在软骨缺口处有平滑肌束和混合性腺。

（2）高倍镜：

1）假复层纤毛柱状上皮由形状不同、高矮不一的细胞组成。细胞界限不清，但可见胞核排列在不同的水平上。上皮表面的纤毛和基底部的基膜明显可见。柱状细胞之间夹有杯状细胞。

2）混合性腺由浆液性腺泡和黏液性腺泡组成，有时可见浆半月。

2. 要求识别

（1）假复层纤毛柱状上皮。

（2）基膜。

（3）固有层。

（4）黏膜下层。

（5）混合性腺。

（6）透明软骨。

肺

（二）肺

1. 染色　HE。

（1）低倍镜：

1）小支气管管壁较厚，管腔较大，其结构与气管基本相似。黏膜上皮为假复层纤毛柱状上皮。固有层薄，外有一层较完整的环形平滑肌。由于平滑肌的收缩，致使黏膜形成皱襞突入管腔，管腔变得不规则。黏膜下层为疏松结缔组织，内含混合性腺，有时腺体伸入外膜。外膜由疏松结缔组织和散在软骨片构成，其中可见小血管的切面。

2）细支气管有肺动脉与其伴行，与小支气管相比具有下列特点：管径更小，管壁更薄；管壁中的软骨和腺体大多消失；管壁中的环层平滑肌逐层增多；黏膜皱襞更加明显。

3）呼吸性细支气管与细支气管相比，具有下列特点：管壁开始出现肺泡直接开口；上皮由单层立方上皮移行为肺泡开口处的单层扁平上皮；固有层结缔组织极薄，含少量的平滑肌；管壁内无杯状细胞，无软骨片和腺体。

4）肺泡管是呼吸性细支气管的延伸，管壁有大量的肺泡开口。相邻肺泡之间的管壁结构少，呈结节状膨大，内含少量结缔组织和平滑肌，表面被覆单层立方上皮或单层扁平上皮。

5）肺泡呈半球囊泡，肺泡壁很薄，表面覆以单层扁平上皮。肺泡占整个肺组织的绝大部分空间。

（2）高倍镜：

1）肺泡表面衬以单层肺泡上皮，无法区分Ⅰ型肺泡细胞和Ⅱ型肺泡细胞，上皮外有少量结缔组织。

2）肺泡隔为相邻肺泡间的结缔组织。内含胶原纤维、网状纤维、大量的弹性纤维和丰富的毛细血管网；可见成纤维细胞、巨噬细胞、少量的肥大细胞和浆细胞。

3）肺泡巨噬细胞体积较大，形态不一，有伪足，胞质内常见被吞噬物。分布在肺泡隔和肺泡腔内的巨噬细胞，常吞有粉尘颗粒，称尘细胞。

4）肺泡管有许多肺泡开口，本身管壁结构较少。在切片中所见的肺泡管断面上，可见相邻肺泡开口之间的肺泡隔呈结节状膨大，内含少量平滑肌。

5）肺泡囊是由几个肺泡共同开口的囊状结构，相邻肺泡开口处没有结节状膨大。

2. 要求识别

（1）小支气管。

（2）细支气管。

（3）呼吸性细支气管。

（4）肺泡管。

（5）肺泡囊。

（6）肺泡。

二、复 习 思 考 题

（1）简述气管的管壁结构特点。

（2）简述肺呼吸性细支气管和肺泡管的结构特点。

（3）简述从气管至终末性细支气管的管壁结构渐变过程。

（4）简述肺泡的结构。

三、图 片 思 考 题

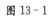
图 13 - 1

图 13 - 2

（黄少萍）

Chapter 13

RESPIRATORY SYSTEM

Learning Points

☞ The morphological structure and the function of the conducting portion of the lung.

☞ The morphological structure and the function of the respiratory portion of the lung.

Part I   Experiment Contents

trachea

1. Trachea

A. Staining   HE.

(1) Low power:

1) The innermost layer of the mucosa is pseudo-stratified ciliated columnar epithelium. It rests on the basement membrane. Under this membrane is the lamina propria which is composed of loose connective tissue containing abundant elastic fibers, glandular ducts, blood vessels, lymphatic tissue and plasma cells.

2) The submucosa consists of loose connective tissue. There is no clear boundary between the lamina propria and the submucosa. The submucosa contains some mixed glands and small blood vessels.

3) The outer layer of the trachea is the adventitia, which contains the hyaline cartilage and loose connective tissue. In this layer, there are C-shaped hyaline cartilage rings. The cartilage gap is covered by the smooth muscle bundles, and mixed glands can also be observed in this area.

(2) High power:

1) Pseudostratified ciliated columnar epithelium is composed of several types of cells with different shapes and heights. The cell boundaries are unclear, the nuclei are visible and found in various levels. The cilia of the epithelial surface and the basement membrane of the epithelium are clearly visible. Goblet cells are scattered between the columnar cells.

2）The mixed glands are composed of serous acini and mucous acini, and sometimes the serous demilunes are visible.

B. Identification requirements

（1）Pseudostratified ciliated columnar epithelium.

（2）Basement membrane.

（3）Lamina propria.

（4）Submucosa.

（5）Mixed gland.

（6）Hyaline cartilage.

lung

2. Lung

A. Staining　HE.

（1）Low power：

1）The wall of the small bronchi is thick，the lumen is large. The structure of its wall is similar to that of the trachea. The mucosa is composed of the pseudostratified ciliated columnar epithelium and the thin lamina propria with a circular layer of smooth muscle beneath it. The contraction of the muscle cells results in mucosal folds projecting into the lumen，and accordingly，the lumen becomes irregular. Submucosa consists of loose connective tissue containing mixed glands which sometimes extend into the adventitia. The adventitia is composed of loose connective tissue containing plates of cartilage and small blood vessels.

2）Compared with the small bronchi，the bronchioles have the following features：the diameter is smaller and the wall is thinner；most of the cartilage and glands in the wall disappear；the smooth muscle relatively increases in the wall, arranged circularly outside the lamina propria；mucosal folds are conspicuous and the lamina propria is thinner.

3）Compared with the bronchioles, respiratory bronchioles have the following features：their wall is interrupted by the openings of the alveoli；the epithelium shifts from simple cuboidal epithelium to simple squamous epithelium which covers the rim of the alveolar openings；the lamina propria is thin，consists of connective tissue and smooth muscle；there are no goblet cells, cartilages or glands in its wall.

4）Alveoli ducts are the distal extensions of the respiratory bronchioles. It's wall contains lots of the opening of alveoli. The remaining wall between the adjacent advoli is less and forms the knobs，which is covered by simple cuboidal or squamous.

5）Alveoli are the polyhedral vesicles and the walls are very thin，their surface covered by simple squamous epithelium. Alveoli constitute the vast majority of the lung tissue.

（2）High power：

1）The surface of alveoli is lined with a single layer of alveolar epithelium and it is difficult to distinguish the two types of cells from each other. Beneath the epithelium is a small amount of connective tissue.

2) The alveolar septum is the connective tissue between adjacent alveoli, containing collagen fibers, reticular fibers, and lots of elastic fibers and rich in capillary network. Moreover, fibroblasts, macrophages, a small amount of mast cells and plasma cells can also be seen in this part.

3) The macrophages are large in volume and different in shape, some have pseudopodia. Their cytoplasm, sometimes contains phagocytotic dust particles. Macrophages, named alveolar dust cells as well, distribute in the lung compartment and alveolar spaces.

4) The alveolar ducts contain numerous openings of alveoli on their wall. The remaining wall between the adjacent alveolar appears as knobs, which contain a small amount of smooth muscle.

5) Alveolar sacs are spaces surrounded by clusters of alveoli. There are no any knobs in the alveolar sacs.

B. Identification requirements

(1) Small bronchi.

(2) Bronchioles.

(3) Respiratory bronchioles.

(4) Alveolar ducts.

(5) Alveolar sacs.

(6) Alveoli.

Part II   Questions for Review

(1) Briefly describe the structural features of the tracheal wall.

(2) Briefly describe the structural features of the respiratory bronchioles and the alveolar duct.

(3) Briefly describe the gradual changes in the wall from the trachea to the terminal bronchioles.

(4) Briefly describe the structural feature of alveoli.

Part III   Pictures Questions for Review

Fig.13 - 1   Fig.13 - 2

(Huang Shaoping)

第十四章

泌 尿 系 统

学习要点

☞ 肾的组织结构。

☞ 肾单位的结构。

☞ 集合管系的结构。

☞ 球旁复合体的结构。

一、实 验 内 容

肾

（一）肾

1. 染色　　HE。

（1）低倍镜：

1）肾表面被覆一层致密结缔组织组成的纤维膜,外有残留的脂肪囊。

2）肾实质可根据位置的深浅及肾小体的有无,来区分皮质和髓质。皮质在外周,内含散在的肾小体和密集的肾小管断面,同时可见由髓质呈辐射状伸入皮质的一些直行管道,染成紫蓝色,即髓放线。位于髓放线之间的皮质称皮质迷路。

3）髓质位于肾的深部,可见到髓袢、集合管、乳头管和许多毛细血管的切面。在皮质和髓质的分界处,还可看到管径比较粗大的弓形血管的断面。

（2）高倍镜：

1）肾小体由毛细血管盘绕而成的血管球和其外面的肾小囊组成。切片中偶见有入球、出球微动脉出入的血管极,或与近曲小管相连的尿极。在切片中,血管球的毛细血管壁不易分辨,可见许多细胞核(包括内皮细胞核、各种白细胞核、球内系膜细胞核、足细胞核等,不必细分)。血管球和肾小囊脏层周围的腔隙为肾小囊腔。肾小囊壁层由单层扁平上皮组成,脏层是足细胞。

2）致密斑由远曲小管靠近肾小体血管极侧的管壁上皮细胞分化而成。管壁上皮细胞增高变窄,形成的椭圆形斑,细胞核卵圆形,染色较深,且排列密集。

3）近端小管的曲部(又称近曲小管)管径大,管腔小而不规则;管壁由单层立方上皮或锥体形细胞围成,胞体大,细胞境界不清,胞质嗜酸性,染成深红色,核圆形,较大,染色略浅,位于基底部,核间距离不等。腔面粗糙不平整,有刷状缘。

4）远曲小管与近曲小管相比：管径小而管腔大;管壁为单层立方上皮,胞质嗜酸性较弱,染色较浅,细胞境界较清楚;核圆形,且位于中央或近腔面。管腔面较平整,无刷状缘。

5）集合小管管径大,管腔也大,上皮为单层立方或单层柱状,细胞质染色浅而清亮,细胞境界清楚。核圆形,位于细胞中部或基底部,染色略深。

6）细段管径小,由单层扁平上皮细胞构成,胞质少且染色淡,核椭圆形突向管腔,此管腔易与毛细血管混淆,与毛细血管的区别是：细段腔内无红细胞;胞质较多;在同一切面上管壁的核数量较多。

2.要求识别

（1）皮质。

（2）髓质。

（3）肾小体。

（4）近曲小管。

（5）细段。

（6）远曲小管。

（7）集合小管。

（8）致密斑。

膀胱

（二）膀胱

1.染色　　HE。

（1）低倍镜：

1）膀胱黏膜向腔内突起形成许多不规则的皱襞,上皮为变移上皮,有6～8层细胞,其表层细胞呈长方形,即盖细胞。固有层由细密的结缔组织组成,含有丰富的血管、神经,其深面的结缔组织较疏松。

2）肌层分为内纵、中环和外纵三层平滑肌,但三层之间分界不明显,肌束之间充填有结缔组织,并有丰富的血管。

3）外膜一部分为浆膜,其余的为疏松结缔组织组成的纤维膜。

（2）高倍镜：

重点观察变移上皮,即变移上皮的层次、结构特点、表面盖细胞的形状,试与复层扁平上皮相比较,有何区别。

2.要求识别

（1）膀胱变移上皮。

（2）盖细胞。

（3）肌层。

（4）外膜。

输尿管

（三）输尿管

1.染色　　HE。

（1）低倍镜：

1）区分输尿管的黏膜、肌层和外膜。

2）与高倍镜观察下的膀胱结构作比较。

（2）高倍镜：

1）黏膜表面衬以变移上皮，上皮下方为少量结缔组织构成的固有层，内含丰富的血管。黏膜形成许多纵行皱襞突向管腔，使管腔横断面呈星状。

2）肌层较厚，上 2/3 由内纵和外环两层平滑肌构成，分界不清。下 1/3 为内纵、中环和外纵三层平滑肌，由于肌纤维走行方向不一致，有时不易区分其层次。

3）外膜为疏松结缔组织构成的纤维膜，内含血管和神经。

2. 要求识别

（1）输尿管的各层结构。

（2）变移上皮的结构特点。

二、复 习 思 考 题

（1）简述肾小体、肾小囊的光镜结构特点。

（2）简述肾小管各段的光镜结构特点。

（3）简述致密斑的结构特点。

（4）简述膀胱变移上皮的结构特点。

三、图 片 思 考 题

图 14-1　　　　图 14-2

（黄少萍）

Chapter 14

URINARY SYSTEM

Learning Points

☞ The structure of the kidney.
☞ The structure of the nephron.
☞ The structure of the collecting tubule system.
☞ The structure of the juxtaglomerular complex.

Part I   Experiment Contents

1. Kidney

kidney

A. Staining   HE.

(1) Low power:

1) Kidney is covered by a thin capsule of dense connective tissue, outside of which is the residual fat sac.

2) The kidney parenchyma is divided into cortex and medulla, both of which can be distinguished from each other according to the location or the presence of renal corpuscle. The cortex is located in the periphery containing scattered renal corpuscles and numerous cross-sections of the renal tubules. Some parallel arrays of tubules projected into the cortex from the medulla are named medullary rays which are stained purple blue. The cortex tissue between the medullary rays is termed cortical labyrinth.

3) Renal medulla is located deeply in the kidney. The medulla contains Henle's loop, collecting tubules, the nipple-like projection or papilla, and many profiles of capillaries. Furthermore, the cross-section of the arcuate blood vessels with large diameter can also be seen at the boundaries of the cortex and medulla.

(2) High power:

1) The renal corpuscle is composed of a tuft of capillaries (called the glomerulus) and the surrounding double-layered epithelial capsule (called Bowman's capsule). Occasionally, the afferent arteriole entering or efferent arteriole leaving the vascular pole, or proximal convoluted tubule connecting to urinary pole can be observed in some area. However, the capillary wall in some sections is not easily distinguished. In

glomerulus many nuclei (including nuclei of the endothelial cells, white blood cells, mesangial cells, podocytes, etc.) can be observed, but there is no need to distinguish each from others. The double-layered epithelial capsule surrounding the glomerulus is the renal capsule. Its parietal layer consists of a simple squamous epithelium, the visceral layer are podocytes not easily to the distinguished.

2) Macula densa is derived from the epithelial cells of the distal convoluted tubule near the renal vascular pole, the epithelial cells become columnar and closely packed together forming a oval disc. The nuclei of the cells are oval, deeply stained and arranged closely.

3) The proximal convoluted tubule is large in diameter, small and irregular in the lumen. The wall of the tubule consists of simple cuboidal or pyramidal cells, the cell body is large with unclear cell boundary. The cytoplasm of the cell is acidophilic and appears as red after staining. The nuclear is round, large, pale-stained, and located in the base part of the cell, the number of nuclei around the lumen is for 4 to 5, and the distances between the nuclei are different. The surface of the lumen is rough because of the brush borders.

4) Compared with the proximal convoluted tubule, the distal convoluted tubule has the following features: The diameter is small, yet the lumen is large. The wall of the tubule is the simple cuboidal epithelium, stained deeply and the cell boundary is clear. The nuclei are round, and arranged regularly and densely. The number of nuclei around the lumen is for 6 to 8, and the distances between the neighbouring nuclei are almost equal. The luminal surface is rather flat owing to no brush borders.

5) The diameter of the collecting tubule is large, and its lumen is large too. The epithelium is simple cuboidal or simple columnar cells, their cytoplasm stained lightly and clearly. Round nuclei are stained slightly dark and located in the middle or base part of the cells.

6) The diameter of the thin segments is small. Its wall consists of a single squamous epithelium containing little cytoplasm and is stained pale. The nucleus is oval and projects a little into the lumen, which is easily confused with the capillaries. Compared with the capillaries, the thin segments have the following features: no erythrocytes in the lumen; more cytoplasm; more nuclei around the lumen on the same section.

B. Identification requirements

(1) Capsule.

(2) Cortex.

(3) Medulla.

(4) Renal corpuscle.

(5) Proximal tubule.

(6) Distal tubule.

(7) Collecting tubule.

(8) Macula densa.

bladder

2. Bladder

A. Staining HE.

(1) Low power:

1) The mucosa of the bladder form many irregular folds. The mucosal epithelium is transitional epithelium containing for 6 to 8 layers of cells, the superficial cells of which are large and round or rectangular. Lamina propria consists of loose-to-dense connective tissue containing plenty of blood vessels, nerves, and lymphoid nodules. The underlying tissue is loose connective tissue.

2) The muscular layer can be divided into internal longitudinal, middle circular, and outer longitudinal layers of smooth muscle, while the boundaries among them are not obvious. Between the neighbouring layers, there is connective tissue rich in blood vessels.

3) The upper part of the bladder is covered externally by an adventitia called serosa, while the remainder is covered by loose connective tissues called fibrous membranes.

(2) High power:

Observe the layers of the transitional epithelium, its structural character istics, and the morphological features of umbrella cells. What is the difference between transitional epithelium and stratified squamous epithelium?

B. Identification requirements

(1) Transitional epithelium.

(2) Tectorial cell.

(3) Muscularis.

(4) Adventitia.

ureter

3. Ureter

A. Staining HE.

(1) Low power:

1) Distinguish the mucosa, muscularis and adventitia of the ureter.

2) Observe and compare the structure of the ureter with that of the bladder under high power.

(2) High power:

1) The surface of mucosa is lined with transitional epithelium, beneath which is the lamina propria composed of a small amount of connective tissue and rich in blood vessels. The mucosa forms many longitudinal folds protruding into the lumen and the lumen appears star-shaped.

2) Muscularis is thick, and its upper two-thirds contains two layers of smooth muscle: the inner longitudinal and outer circular layer. The lower one-third is composed of inner longitudinal, middle circular and outer longitudinal layers of smooth muscle. Owing to the inconsistent directions of the muscle fibers, it is difficult to distinguish every layer clearly sometimes.

3) The adventitia is a thin layer of loose connective tissues called fibrous membrane containing blood vessels and nerves fibers.

B. Identification requirements

(1) Structure of each layer of the ureter.

(2) Transitional epithelium.

Part II   Questions for Review

(1) Briefly describe the structure of the renal corpuscle and Bowman's capsule.

(2) Briefly describe the structure of different segments of the renal tubules.

(3) Briefly describe the structure of the macula densa.

(4) Briefly describe the structure of the epithelium of the bladder.

Part III   Pictures Questions for Review

Fig.14 - 1   Fig.14 - 2

(Huang Shaoping)

第十五章

内 分 泌 系 统

学习要点

☞ 内分泌腺的一般结构,两类内分泌细胞的结构特点及分布。
☞ 甲状腺和甲状旁腺的光镜、电镜结构特点及分泌激素。
☞ 肾上腺的光镜、电镜结构特点及分泌激素。
☞ 脑垂体的一般结构和分部,腺垂体各部和神经垂体的结构特点、激素来源。垂体门脉系统的组成及其功能意义。下丘脑与腺垂体及神经垂体的关系。
☞ 弥散神经内分泌系统的概念和意义。

一、实 验 内 容

甲状腺

(一) 甲状腺

1. 染色　　HE。

(1) 低倍镜:

1) 甲状腺外有薄层结缔组织构成的被膜,被膜伸入腺实质。

2) 腺实质中有大量含有红色胶质的甲状腺滤泡,大小不等,圆形或卵圆形。

3) 滤泡间为结缔组织和血管,以及滤泡间细胞团。

(2) 高倍镜:

1) 甲状腺滤泡上皮细胞一般为单层立方上皮,细胞境界清楚。

2) 滤泡上皮细胞根据其功能状态不同,可分为矮柱状或立方形,滤泡腔内为红染均质的胶质。

3) 滤泡旁细胞位于滤泡基膜上,散在嵌于滤泡上皮细胞之间,或二三成群分布于滤泡间,体积大,胞质透亮、着色浅,核圆形。

2. 要求识别

(1) 甲状腺滤泡上皮。

(2) 胶质。

(3) 滤泡旁细胞。

甲状旁腺

（二）甲状旁腺

1. 染色　　HE。

（1）低倍镜：

1）外有薄层的结缔组织被膜。

2）腺实质为密集的腺细胞排列成团或相互吻合的索，呈紫蓝色。

（2）高倍镜：

1）主细胞数量最多，体积小，胞体圆或卵圆形，核小圆形居中而胞质浅亮，细胞排列成不规则条索，并相互吻合，周围可见少量结缔组织。

2）腺细胞之间见许多毛细血管。

3）嗜酸性细胞单个或成群分布于主细胞之间，细胞较大，核小，胞质嗜酸性。

2. 要求识别　　甲状旁腺主细胞。

肾上腺

（三）肾上腺

1. 染色　　HE。

（1）低倍镜：

1）肾上腺表面有结缔组织被膜，其外方有脂肪组织和血管。

2）被膜下染成紫红色的细胞索团是皮质，自外向中心分为球状带、束状带和网状带，之间无截然分界。

3）在皮质深部，腺体中央是髓质，其中含有几个较大而不规则的腔，是中央静脉及其属支。

（2）高倍镜：

1）球状带紧靠被膜下，此带最薄，细胞排列成团。胞体较小、圆形或卵圆形，核圆、着色深。

2）束状带位于球状带深层，占皮质大部分，细胞排列成单行或双行的细胞束，细胞大，多边形，泡沫状。血窦位于细胞束之间，近网状带处细胞排列不规则。

3）网状带与束状带无明显界限，而与髓质分界参差不齐，此带较窄，细胞交错成网，血窦呈不规则裂隙状。细胞小而着色红。

4）髓质主要由嗜铬细胞组成，胞质嗜碱性。细胞排列成团、索状，其间有血窦及少量结缔组织。髓质中还有腔大而管壁厚薄不均的中央静脉及属支。

2. 要求识别

（1）球状带。

（2）束状带。

（3）网状带。

（4）髓质嗜铬细胞。

脑垂体

（四）脑垂体

1. 染色　　HE。

（1）低倍镜：

1）表面有结缔组织被膜，内有许多血管断面。

2）远侧部含有大量染成红色或紫红色细胞。

3）神经部着色浅,含有许多无髓神经纤维和神经胶质细胞。

4）中间部较窄,可见几个大小不一的滤泡。

（2）高倍镜：

1）远侧部：仔细辨认嗜酸性细胞（胞质中有粉红色颗粒）、嗜碱性细胞（胞体大,数量少）及嫌色细胞（数量最多,胞体小,浅染,界限不清）。细胞索团之间为血窦。

2）中间部：由几个大小不一的滤泡及少量嗜碱性细胞构成。

3）神经部：有无髓神经纤维及垂体细胞,核圆或卵圆形,核周可见少量胞质,但突起不可见。有的细胞中含有棕褐色色素。神经纤维浅红色,纤维间有散在分布的浅红色均质状小体,即赫林体,此外尚有血窦及少量结缔组织细胞。

2. 要求识别

（1）远侧部各种细胞。

（2）中间部。

（3）神经部：垂体细胞、无髓神经纤维、赫林体。

二、复 习 思 考 题

（1）简述甲状腺的两种组成细胞及其结构特点。

（2）简述肾上腺皮质的微细结构和功能特点。

（3）简述垂体的结构特点。

三、图 片 思 考 题

图 15-1

图 15-2

图 15-3

（王　晖）

Chapter 15

ENDOCRINE SYSTEM

Learning Points

☞ The general structure of the endocrine glands, the structural characteristics and distribution of the two kinds of endocrine cells.

☞ The structural characteristics of thyroid and parathyroid glands under light and electron microscope as well as their secreted hormones.

☞ The structural characteristics of adrenal gland under light and electron microscope, and its secreted hormones.

☞ The general structure of the pituitary gland (hypophysis) and its partition, the structural features of adenohypophysis and neurohypophysis and the source of hormones. The composition and functional significance of the hypophyseal portal system as well as the relationship among the hypothalamus, adenohypophysis and neurohypophysis.

☞ The concept and the significance of the diffused neuroendocrine system (APUD system).

Part I   Experiment Contents

thyroid gland

1. Thyroid gland

A. Staining   HE.

(1) Low power:

1) The gland is covered by a loose connective tissue capsule that sends septa into the parenchyma.

2) Note the prominent histologic features of the parenchyma: numerous colloid-containing follicles of various sizes, round or oval in shape.

3) The connective tissue with blood vessels and small isolated clusters of cells are frequently identified between the thyroid follicles.

(2) High power:

1) The thyroid gland consists of follicles lined by a single low cuboidal epithelium, and the outline of cells is clear.

2) The follicular cells may be low cuboidal or low columnar according to their function, and enclose a central lumen filled with red-stained colloid.

3) The parafollicular cells or, are situated on the basement membrane, scattered and interspersed among follicular cells or in clusters between follicles. These cells are large with transparent and pale-staining cytoplasm and a round nucleus.

B. Identification requirements

(1) Follicular epithelial cells.

(2) Colloid.

(3) Parafollicular cells.

2. Parathyroid glands

parathyroid
glands

A. Staining　　HE.

(1) Low power:

1) Each parathyroid gland is surrounded by an extremely thin connective tissue capsule.

2) The parenchyma of the gland consists of densely packed clusters or anatomizing cords of gland cells, which are stained purple-blue.

(2) High power:

1) The majority of cells with small centrally placed round nuclei and clear cytoplasm are chief cells, which form irregular, anastomosing cords supported by delicate connective tissue.

2) Capillaries are abundant between the glandular cells.

3) Oxyphil cells are distributed among the chief cells as single cells or small groups with a larger cell body, small nucleus, and eosinophilic cytoplasm.

B. Identification requirements　　Chief cells.

3. Adrenal glands

adrenal
glands

A. Staining　　HE.

(1) Low power:

1) The gland is surrounded by a thick connective tissue capsule, with adipose tissue and blood vessels outside the capsule.

2) Beneath the capsule is the cortex, which is stained red-violet. The cortex consists of three concentric zones which, from the surface inwards, are termed the zona glomerulosa, the zona fasciculata and the zona reticularis. There are no clear boundaries among these three zones.

3) Medulla is located in the central part of the gland where some large and irregular cavities of central vein and its branches are found.

(2) High power:

1) The zona glomerulosa closely adjoins the capsule and is the thinnest zona. Cells

of zona glomerulosa are small, round or oval and arranged in spherical groups. Their nuclei are dark and round.

2）The zona fasciculata is beneath the zona glomerulosa and occupies most of the cortex. The cells are large, polyhedral, and spongy arranged in single or double lines. Between cellular cords lies sinusoid, and the cells near the zona reticularis are irregularly arranged.

3）Zona reticularis has no sharp dividing line with zona fasciculata, but a clear and irregular one with medulla. This zona is narrow and their cells are typically smaller, and red-stained, forming the anastomosing cords. Sinusoids are irregular slit-like.

4）Medulla is mainly composed of chromaffin cells. The cytoplasm is weakly basophilic. The cells are arranged in clumps and cords, separated by sinusoids and some connective tissue. In the medulla the central vein and its branches are obvious.

B. Identification requirements

（1）Zona glomerulosa.

（2）Zona fasciculata.

（3）Zona reticularis.

（4）Chromaffin cells.

pituitary
gland
（hypophysis）

4. Pituitary gland (hypophysis)

A. Staining   HE.

（1）Low power：

1）The gland is surrounded by a thick connective tissue capsule with numerous blood vessels in.

2）The glandular cells in the pars distalis are stained red or amaranthine.

3）The neurohypophysis is lightly stained and consists of a mass of unmyelinated axons of secretory nerve cells and glial cells.

4）The pars intermedia is narrow and several follicles of different sizes are found.

（2）High power：

1）Pars distalis：Try to distinguish the three basic cell types：acidophils (cytoplasm is filled with pink granules), basophils (less numerous, large in size), chromophobes (unstained or weakly stained, small in size, most numerous, outline is unclear). Note also the extensive network of blood-filled sinusoids surrounding these endocrine cells.

2）Pars intermedia：It is made up of weakly basophilic cells and contains a few follicles varied in size.

3）Pars nervosa：Unmyelinated nerve fibers and pituicytes are found. The pituicytes have round or oval nuclei with a small amount of cytoplasm around them, however, their processes are invisible. Some cells contain brown pigments. The nerve fibers are light red, among which small light red bodies called Herring bodies are distributed. Besides, the sinusoids and a few connective tissue cells are also visible.

B. Identification requirements

(1) Different cell types in pars distalis.

(2) Pars intermedia.

(3) Pars nervosa: pituicytes unmyelinated nerve fibres, and Herring bodies.

Part II Questions for Review

(1) Briefly describe the structural features of two main cells in the thyroid gland.

(2) Briefly describe the structural and functional characteristics of the cortex of the adrenal gland.

(3) Briefly describe the structural features of the hypophysis.

Part III Pictures Questions for Review

Fig.15 - 1   Fig.15 - 2   Fig.15 - 3

(Wang Hui)

第十六章

男性生殖系统

学习要点

☞ 睾丸的一般结构。
☞ 生精小管的结构和功能。精子发生的过程。
☞ 睾丸间质细胞的结构与功能。
☞ 附睾与输精管的结构特点与功能。
☞ 前列腺的结构特点与功能。

一、实验内容

睾丸

（一）睾丸

1. 染色　　HE。

（1）低倍镜：

1）白膜位于睾丸表面，由致密结缔组织构成。其内面是富含血管的疏松结缔组织。

2）睾丸背侧结缔组织增厚称睾丸纵隔，伸入睾丸实质并形成小隔，将实质分成许多小叶。

3）生精小管是睾丸的主要成分。数量很多，切片上呈圆形或卵圆形。管壁由生精上皮构成，为多层大小不一的圆形细胞。

4）生精小管之间有少量结缔组织称睾丸间质。

（2）高倍镜：

1）生精小管基膜明显，基膜外有胶原纤维和1～2层肌样细胞。生精上皮细胞分支持细胞和生精细胞。

2）支持细胞数量少，体积大，锥体形，单个分散在生精细胞之间。细胞境界不清。胞核多位于初级精母细胞和精原细胞之间，体积大，圆形、三角形或不规则形，着色浅，核仁明显。

3）生精细胞排列成多层。从近基膜向管腔方向发育逐渐成熟，依次分为精原细胞、初级精母细胞、次级精母细胞、精子细胞和精子五种不同发育阶段。① 精原细胞靠近基膜，胞体较小，呈圆形，核圆形，着色深，可见核仁。② 初级精母细胞在精原细胞的内侧，有 2～3 层细胞,胞体较精原细胞大,圆形或卵圆形。核大,常呈分裂象,染色质排列成丝球状。③ 次级精母细胞因存在时间短,在切片中很难看到。④ 精子细胞近管腔,有多层细胞。胞体最小,呈圆形,胞质少,核小着色略深。⑤ 蝌蚪形的精子在近腔面或管腔中。头部胞核变长,染色深,插在支持细胞内,尾部细长朝向管腔。

4) 间质细胞单个或三五成群分布在生精小管之间的结缔组织中,胞体较大,圆形或多边形,胞质嗜酸性,核大而圆,着色浅。

2. **要求识别**

(1) 生精小管。

(2) 生精细胞。

(3) 支持细胞。

(4) 间质细胞。

(二) 附睾

附睾

1. **染色**　　HE。

(1) 低倍镜:

1) 附睾由多条输出小管和 1 条长且高度弯曲的附睾管组成。

2) 输出小管管径较细,腔型不规则。

3) 附睾管管径较大,管壁较厚,管腔规则。

(2) 高倍镜:

1) 输出小管管壁上皮由低柱状细胞和高柱状纤毛细胞分群相间排列而成,腔面起伏不平。基膜外有少量平滑肌环绕。

2) 附睾管由假复层柱状上皮构成,腔型规则,上皮细胞表面有许多粗长的静纤毛。腔内有精子和分泌物。基膜外有薄层平滑肌。

2. **要求识别**

(1) 输出小管。

(2) 附睾管。

(三) 输精管

输精管

1. **染色**　　HE。

(1) 低倍镜:

1) 输精管由黏膜、肌层和外膜组成。

2) 黏膜很薄,有纵行皱襞。

3) 肌层很厚,分内纵、中环、外纵三层平滑肌。

4) 外膜较薄,由结缔组织构成。

(2) 高倍镜:

1) 黏膜由假复层柱状上皮和薄层结缔组织固有层构成。少数上皮细胞表面有细长的静纤毛。

2) 肌层内纵肌较薄,中环肌和外纵肌较厚。

3) 外膜为纤维膜。疏松结缔组织中含有许多血管和少数无髓神经纤维。

2. 要求识别

(1) 黏膜上皮。

(2) 肌层。

(3) 外膜。

前列腺

(四) 前列腺

1. 染色　　HE。

(1) 低倍镜:

1) 被膜较厚,由富含弹性纤维结缔组织和平滑肌构成,伸入腺组织之间形成间隔,分隔成许多小叶。

2) 被膜中含有许多血管和神经断面,有的可见成群分布的、被染成紫蓝色的、大的多边形细胞是副交感神经节细胞。

3) 前列腺为复管泡状腺,其分泌部腔较大有皱襞,故腔型不规则。

4) 前列腺腺腔中有被染成粉红色圆形的前列腺凝固体。

(2) 高倍镜:

1) 前列腺分泌部的上皮形态不一,为单层立方柱状及假复层柱状上皮。上皮及其下面的结缔组织隆起形成高低不等的皱襞。

2) 凝固体为嗜酸性的同心圆板层状。

3) 在结缔组织间隔中含有大量平滑肌,并有血管和无髓神经纤维。

2. 要求识别

(1) 被膜。

(2) 前列腺分泌部。

(3) 腺上皮。

(4) 凝固体。

二、复 习 思 考 题

(1) 简述睾丸支持细胞的结构及功能特点。

(2) 简述生精小管的结构特点。

(3) 简述血-睾屏障的分层结构及功能特点。

三、图 片 思 考 题

图 16-1

图 16-2

图 16-3

(王　蕾)

Chapter 16

MALE REPRODUCTIVE SYSTEM

Learning Points

☞ The general structure of the testis.

☞ The structure and function of the seminiferous tubule; the process of spermatogenesis.

☞ The structure and function of Leydig cells.

☞ The structural features and function of the epididymis and ductus deferens.

☞ The structural characteristics and function of the prostate.

Part I   Experiment Contents

testis

1. Testis

A. Staining   HE.

(1) Low power:

1) Each testis is surrounded by the tunica albuginea, a thick capsule of dense connective tissue rich in blood vessels in the inner layer.

2) The connective tissue is thickened on the posterior surface of the testis to form the mediastinum testis, from which fibrous septa penetrate into the gland and form wedge-shaped lobules.

3) Within each lobule seminiferous tubules are tightly packed with numerous round or oval profiles, and its luminal surface is lined by seminiferous epithelium which is composed of several layers of round cells of different sizes.

4) The spaces between the seminiferous tubules are filled with interstitium composed of connective tissue.

(2) High power:

1) The outer surface of the seminiferous tubules is enclosed by a well-defined basal lamina which is surrounded with one to two layers of myoid cells. The seminiferous epithelium contains Sertoli and spermatogenic cells.

2) The Sertoli cells are elongated pyramid cells distributed among spermatogenic cells. Their nuclei are located between the spermatogonial cells and the primary

spermatocytes，nucleus is large，triangular or irregular in shape and lightly stained with a prominent nucleolus.

3）The spermatogenic cells are made up of several layers of cells，which are divided into spermatogonia，primary spermatocytes，secondary spermatocytes，spermatids and sperms from the basal lamina to the luminal surface of the seminiferous tubules. ① Spermatogonia just rest on the basal lamina. The cell is relatively small in shape，with a round and darkly stained nucleus containing a prominent nucleolus. ② Primary spermatocytes lie in the middle layer of the epithelium，at the internal side of the spermatogonia，and usually for 2 to 3 layers. The cell is round or oval in shape and is larger than spermatogonia. The nuclei are large with thread-like chromosomes. The mitotic figures are easy seen. ③ Secondary spermatocytes are rare in histological sections because they undergo the second meiotic division almost immediately after being formed. ④ Spermatids are small cells with dark heterochromatic nuclei located next to the lumen. ⑤ Spermatozoa are tadpole in shape，their darkly stained heads appear to insert into the Sertoli cells and their long and thin tails are left free in the lumen.

4）Leydig cells are large round cells gathered in groups and located in the interstitial tissue between the seminiferous tubules，their cytoplasm are strongly acidophilic，and their nuclei are large，round and lightly stained.

B. Identification requirements

（1）Seminiferous tubules.

（2）Spermatogenic cells.

（3）Sertoli cells.

（4）Leydig cells.

epididymis

2. Epididymis

A. Staining　　HE.

（1）Low power：

1）It is comprised of several efferent ductules and a long，coiled epididymal duct.

2）Efferent ductules are of small size，and their lumen is irregular.

3）The epididymal duct is larger in diameter and has a thick wall and a regular lumen.

（2）High power：

1）The epithelium of efferent ductules is composed of alternating groups of cuboidal and columnar cells which are often ciliated. The epithelium is bounded by a few of circularly arranged smooth fibers.

2）The epididymal duct is lined by a very tall pseudostratified columnar epithelium with long stereocilia，their basal lamina is surrounded by a thin layer of smooth muscle cells，and the spermatozoa and secretion are stored in the lumen.

B. Identification requirements

(1) Efferent ductules.

(2) Epididymal duct.

3. Ductus deferens

A. Staining　HE.

(1) Low power:

1) Its wall is divided into three layers: mucosa, muscularis and

ductus
deferens

adventitia.

2) The mucosa is thin and forms longitudinal plica.

3) The muscularis is thick and subdivided into three layers of smooth muscle fibers: the inner longitudinal layer, the middle circular layer and the outer longitudinal layer.

4) The adventitia is composed of connective tissue.

(2) High power:

1) The mucosa consists of a pseudostratified columnar epithelium and a thin layer of loose connective tissue, and long stereocilia are found on the surface of some of the epithelial cells.

2) The muscularis is well developed and consists of a thin longitudinal, a thick middle circular and outer longitudinal layers of smooth muscle.

3) The adventitia is fibrosa containing numerous blood vessels and a few unmyelinated nerve fibers.

B. Identification requirements

(1) The epithelium of mucosa.

(2) The muscularis.

(3) The adventitia.

4. Prostate gland

A. Staining　HE.

(1) Low power:

1) The prostate gland is covered by a fibro-elastic capsule rich in

prostate
gland

smooth muscle fibers, and the septa from the capsule penetrate into the gland and divide it into lobules.

2) Within the capsule, there are nerves, blood vessels and also some large polyhedral dark purple-stained cells gathering in groups which are parasympathetic ganglion cells.

3) The prostate is a collection of many compound tubule-alveolar glands. The secretory alveoli of the prostate are irregular and vary greatly in size and shape because the folds project into the lumen of the alveoli.

4）The prostatic concretions are round eosinophilic bodies in the secretory alveoli.

（2）High power：

1）The epithelium varies from simple cuboidal or columnar to pseudostratified columnar. The epithelium and underlying connective tissue form folds in various shapes and sizes，which project into the lumen of the secretary alveoli.

2）The eosinophilic prostatic concretions are in the form of concentric lamellae.

3）The glands are embedded into a fibromuscular stroma，which mainly consist of smooth muscles，blood vessels and unmyelinated nerve fibers.

B. Identification requirements

（1）The capsule of the prostate gland.

（2）The secretory alveoli.

（3）The epithelium of the secretory alveoli.

（4）The prostatic concretions.

Part II   Questions for Review

（1）Briefly describe the structure and function of the Sertoli cell.

（2）Briefly describe the structure of the seminiferous tubule.

（3）Briefly describe the structure and function of the blood-testis barrier.

Part III   Pictures Questions for Review

Fig.16 - 1   Fig.16 - 2   Fig.16 - 3

（Wang Lei）

第十七章

女性生殖系统

学习要点

☞ 卵巢的一般结构,各级卵泡及黄体的结构特点。
☞ 子宫的一般结构,子宫内膜的周期性变化。
☞ 输卵管的结构特点。

一、实 验 内 容

卵巢

(一)卵巢

1. 染色　　HE。

(1)低倍镜:

1)表面上皮:位于卵巢表面,由单层扁平或立方细胞覆盖。

2)白膜:位于上皮下方,由致密结缔组织构成,细胞多,纤维少。

3)皮质:由各级卵泡、黄体和富含基质细胞等的较致密的结缔组织组成。各级卵泡由中央一个大的卵母细胞和周围许多卵泡细胞组成。卵巢由浅表向深部依次可以观察到:原始卵泡、初级卵泡、次级卵泡和各种闭锁卵泡。未见成熟卵泡。由于切面关系,有的次级卵泡只见卵泡壁和卵泡腔,而未见到卵母细胞。

4)髓质:由疏松结缔组织构成,含有丰富的血管和一些神经纤维。有的标本一侧有较多的结缔组织和血管,此为卵巢门部。

(2)高倍镜:

1)原始卵泡:在被膜下皮质密集排列,体积最小,由中央一个大的初级卵母细胞和周围一层扁平的卵泡细胞构成。初级卵母细胞的胞质嗜酸性,核大、着色浅,呈空泡状,核仁明显。

2)初级卵泡:体积较原始卵泡大,由中央一个更大的初级卵母细胞和周围单层立方或多层卵泡细胞构成。在初级卵母细胞的外面有一层嗜酸性均质膜称透明带。

3)次级卵泡:体积更大,卵泡细胞层数增多,可达6～12层。在卵泡细胞之间出现卵泡液和卵泡腔。初级卵母细胞及其周围的一些卵泡细胞突入卵泡腔称卵丘。卵泡腔周围的卵泡细胞称颗粒细胞。紧靠透明带的一层卵泡细胞为柱状,呈放射状排列,称放射冠。卵泡外面有结缔组织构成的卵泡膜,卵泡膜分内外两层,内层有膜细胞,富有血管,外层纤维多。

4）闭锁卵泡：卵母细胞退化溶解，透明带皱缩塌陷并可单独保留在结缔组织之中，卵泡细胞溶解。有些卵泡膜内层膜细胞肥大呈多边形，胞质嗜酸性，充满脂滴，被结缔组织分隔成团索状，称间质腺。

5）黄体：是体积很大的细胞团，着色浅。黄体外有结缔组织膜，黄体细胞分两种：① 粒黄体细胞位于中央，占黄体大部分，细胞很多，胞体较大呈多边形，胞质着色浅，充满脂滴而溶解呈空泡状。② 膜黄体细胞位于黄体周围，细胞少，胞体较小，胞质着色较深。黄体中有丰富的毛细血管。

2. 要求识别

（1）表面上皮。

（2）白膜。

（3）原始卵泡。

（4）初级卵泡。

（5）次级卵泡。

（6）闭锁卵泡。

（7）黄体。

子宫

（二）子宫

1. 染色　　HE。

（1）低倍镜：由内向外依次观察子宫壁结构。

1）子宫内膜：即黏膜，由单层柱状上皮和结缔组织固有层组成。子宫内膜大体分为近浅表较厚的功能层和近肌层较薄且着色较深的基底层。固有层中有大量弯曲而扩大的子宫腺。在固有层中自深层直至浅表可见成串的小动脉断面是螺旋动脉。

2）肌层：为很厚的平滑肌，肌层可分三层，但分界不清。此外还含有丰富的血管。

3）外膜：为很薄的结缔组织，外覆有一层间皮的浆膜。

（2）高倍镜：重点观察分泌期子宫内膜。

1）上皮：单层柱状，少数是纤毛细胞，多数是无纤毛的分泌细胞。

2）固有层：结缔组织中细胞多纤维少，基质细胞变肥大，呈圆形或多边形，胞质着色浅，核大而着色浅。结缔组织中含丰富的血管。

3）子宫腺：为管状腺，腺体明显弯曲，腺腔大，腔型不规则，腔内有许多分泌物。腺上皮为单层柱状，可见核上空泡。

4）螺旋动脉：呈自深层直至浅表的成串小动脉结构。

2. 要求识别

（1）子宫壁的三层结构。

（2）子宫上皮。

（3）子宫腺。

（4）螺旋动脉。

输卵管

（三）输卵管

1. 染色　　HE。

（1）低倍镜：管壁由内向外分为黏膜、肌层和外膜三层。

1）黏膜：由单层柱状上皮和固有层构成。黏膜向管腔突出形成许多有分支的纵行皱襞，管腔形态极不规则。

2）肌层：较薄，分内环外纵两层，但分界不清。

3）外膜：疏松结缔组织，内含丰富的血管，外有一层间皮。

（2）高倍镜：主要观察黏膜结构。

1）上皮：为单层柱状上皮，细胞分为纤毛细胞和分泌细胞两种，其中纤毛细胞占多数。

2）固有层：疏松结缔组织，含有丰富的血管和少量散在的平滑肌。

2. 要求识别

（1）输卵管的三层结构。

（2）黏膜上皮和皱襞。

二、复习思考题

（1）比较各个不同发育阶段卵泡的结构特点。

（2）简述黄体的结构和功能。

（3）简述子宫内膜的周期性变化及其激素调节。

（4）简述输卵管的构造。

三、图片复习题

图 17-1

图 17-2

图 17-3

（黄晓燕）

Chapter 17

FEMALE REPRODUCTIVE SYSTEM

Learning Points

☞ The general structure of the ovary, structural features of follicles and corpus luteum.

☞ The general structure of the uterus; cyclical changes of endometrium during menstrual cycle.

☞ The structural characteristics of the uterine tube (oviduct).

Part I Experiment Contents

ovary

1. Ovary

A. Staining   HE.

(1) Low power:

1) The surface of the ovary is covered by a single layer of flat or cuboidal epithelium, called germinal epithelium.

2) Fibrous connective tissue with few fibers and more cell elements form a thin capsule, the tunica albuginea, just beneath the epithelium.

3) The cortical stroma is composed of dense connective tissue containing a great number of follicles of different stages and the corpus luteum. Ovarian follicles consist of one central oocyte and surrounding follicular cells, located from superficial to deep part of the ovary. The following follicles of specific stages are observed: primordial follicles, primary follicles, secondary follicles and atretic follicles. Mature follicles are difficult to observe. In some secondary follicles, only the follicle wall and follicle cavity can be found, the oocyte is not visible because the section is different.

4) The medulla of the ovary is composed of loose connective tissue rich in blood vessels and nerves. For some specimen, the hilus of the ovary containing loose connective tissue and blood vessels are observed on one side of the ovary.

(2) High power:

1) Primordial follicle: It is located in the cortex just beneath tunica albuginea, composed of one central primary oocyte and one layer of squamous follicular cells

outside. The plasma of the oocyte is eosinophilic, and its nucleus is large, vesicular and pale-stained with a prominent nucleolus.

2) Primary follicle: It becomes larger than the primordial follicle. It is composed of a central primary oocyte surrounded by a single or multiple layers of cuboidal or columnar follicular cells. The zona pellucida is observed as a thick homogeneous acidophilic membrane between the oocyte and the follicular cells.

3) Secondary follicle: It continues to enlarge, and the layers of follicular cells (granulosa cells) reach about 6 to 12. Small fluid-filled spaces become visible between the follicular cells, and then these spaces enlarge and fuse to form the follicular antrum. Within the follicular antrum, cumulus oophorus is found which is formed by several layers of follicular cells and a primary oocyte. One layer of radially disposed and columnar granulosa cells attached to zona pellucida is the corona radiata. The theca is divided into the theca interna, rich in capillaris, and the theca externa, which is a fibrous layer.

4) Atretic follicle: The primary oocyte degenerates and dissolves. The zona pellucida becomes wavy and collapsed and may remain alone in the connective tissue. The follicular cells also dissolve. Some thecal cells become polyhedral, filled with lipid droplets, and are divided by connective tissue into clusters forming interstitial gland.

5) Corpus luteum: It is a mass of cells of light color and surrounded by connective tissue. It is formed by both granulosa lutein cells and theca lutein cells. The granulosa lutein cells are the predominant and largest cell type, filled with lipid droplets, vacuolated and located in the center of the corpus lutein. While the theca lutein cells are smaller in size, fewer in number, and located on the periphery of granulose lutein cells. The center of corpus luteum is highly vascularized.

B. Identification requirements

(1) Germinal epithelium.

(2) Tunica albuginea.

(3) Primordial follicles.

(4) Primary follicles.

(5) Secondary follicles.

(6) Atretic follicles.

(7) Corpus luteum.

2. Uterus

uterus

A. Staining   HE.

(1) Low power: Observe three sublayers of the uterine wall.

1) Endometrium: The mucosa consists of simple columnar epithelium and an underlying thick cellular lamina propria. It is divided into two layers, the thicker, more superficial stratum functionalis and the deeper basal

layer, the stratum basale. There are many winding and enlarged uterine glands, and continuous cross sections of spiral arteries are observed in the lamina propria.

2) Myometrium: It consists of interlacing bundles of smooth muscle separated by connective tissue. Three layers may be distinguished, but their boundaries are not clear.

3) Perimetrium: It is a serosa which is composed of a thin layer of loose connective tissue lined by mesothelium.

(2) High power: Focus on secretory phase endometrium.

1) Epithelium: It is simple columnar epithelium with a few ciliated cells and more secretory cells.

2) Lamina propria: It is formed by connective tissue with few fibers but more cells and rich in blood vessels. The hypertrophic stromal cells are round or polygonal, with pale stained cytoplasm and large nucleus.

3) Uterine glands: They are simple tubular glands. They increase in length and become convoluted with dilated lumen. The basal region of granular cells contains accumulated glycogen which was dissolved during slide preparation, thus a vacuolated appearance is visible above the nucleus.

4) Spiral arteries: continuous cross sections of small arteries are observed from the deep to the superficial part of the endometrium.

B. Identification requirements

(1) Uterine wall structure.

(2) Epithelium of uterus.

(3) Uterine glands.

(4) Spiral arteries.

uterine tube (oviduct)

3. Uterine tube (oviduct)

A. Staining　HE.

(1) Low power: the wall of oviduct is divided into three layers from inside to outside: mucosa, muscularis and external serosa.

1) Mucosa: It is composed of simple columnar epithelium and the lamina propria rich in cellular components. The mucosa presents several longitudinal folds, resulting in the formation of the irregular lumen.

2) Muscularis: The smooth muscle bundles are so loosely arranged that it is difficult to clearly define the inner circular and the outer longitudinal layers.

3) Serosa: It is a thin layer of loose connective tissue with numerous blood vessels and covered by mesothelium on the outer surface.

(2) High power: Focus on mucosa.

1) Epithelium: It is simple columnar epithelium with a few secretory cells and more ciliated cells.

2) Lamina propria: It is made up of connective tissue with a few scattered smooth muscle fibers but more blood vessels.

B. Identification requirements

(1) Three layers of the uterine tube.

(2) Epithelium and mucosal folds.

Part II   Questions for Review

(1) Compare the differences in structure of follicle in different stage.

(2) Briefly describe the structural features of corpus luteam and its related function.

(3) Briefly describe the cyclic changes of endometrium and its hormonal regulation.

(4) Briefly describe the structure of the oviduct.

Part III   Pictures Questions for Review

Fig.17 - 1   Fig.17 - 2   Fig.17 - 3

(Huang Xiaoyan)

第十八章

眼 和 耳

学习要点

☞ 眼球壁的结构。

☞ 角膜的结构,角膜缘的特点及巩膜静脉窦的意义。虹膜、睫状体和脉络膜的结构和功能。

☞ 视网膜的结构和功能,黄斑和视神经乳头的结构和意义。

☞ 内耳骨迷路和膜迷路的结构。

☞ 壶腹嵴、椭圆囊斑和球囊斑的结构和功能。螺旋器的结构和功能。

一、实 验 内 容

眼球

(一) 眼球

1. 染色　　HE。

(1) 低倍镜:

1) 眼球壁由三层膜构成:外层的纤维膜、中层的血管膜和内层的视网膜。

2) 眼球前方染成粉红色的角膜为纤维膜的前 1/6,连在角膜后方染成浅红色的巩膜为纤维膜的后 5/6。

3) 在巩膜内侧可见富含色素细胞的脉络膜,脉络膜向前方延续为睫状体和虹膜。

4) 在虹膜后方有染成红色的晶状体。

5) 在脉络膜的内侧为视网膜,个别部位有制片造成的剥脱现象。

(2) 高倍镜:

1) 角膜:自外向内分为:角膜上皮、前界膜、角膜基质、后界膜、角膜内皮。

2) 巩膜:由致密结缔组织构成。在巩膜和角膜移行处的稍内侧有 1～2 个略大的腔隙,内衬一层内皮,即巩膜静脉窦。

3) 虹膜:前面为不连续的成纤维细胞和色素细胞构成的前缘层。中间为含有血管及色素细胞的疏松结缔组织。后面是由两层色素细胞组成的虹膜上皮。

4) 睫状体:位于虹膜后方,切面呈三角形肥厚。前面有许多小突起叫睫状突。

5) 脉络膜:位于巩膜和视网膜之间,由疏松结缔组织构成,内含丰富的血管和色素细胞。

6）视网膜：紧贴脉络膜内面，常因制片过程引起收缩而与脉络膜相脱离。由外向内可依次识别视网膜的四层细胞，即色素上皮层、视细胞层、双极细胞层和节细胞层。在视网膜后方，有视神经盘（又称视神经乳头），此处有视神经和血管出入眼球壁，无感光细胞，为生理性盲点。

2.要求识别

（1）角膜。

（2）巩膜。

（3）睫状体。

（4）视网膜。

（5）视盘。

（二）内耳

内耳

1.染色　　HE。

（1）低倍镜：

1）主要观察耳蜗，由骨组织构成。

2）中央有锥形的骨性蜗轴，轴的两侧有骨性蜗管的横断面。

3）骨性蜗管中有三个小管，上方的腔是前庭阶，下方的腔是鼓室阶，中间的腔是蜗管；前庭阶与蜗管之间是前庭膜；而鼓室阶与蜗管之间是基底膜。

（2）高倍镜：

1）蜗管有以下结构特点：上壁是前庭膜，为斜行的薄层结缔组织膜，两面均为单层扁平上皮，其中一层来自前庭阶，另一层源自蜗管；外壁称血管纹，位于螺旋韧带表面，为含有毛细血管的复层柱状上皮；下壁由骨螺旋板的外侧份和基底膜组成，螺旋器位于基底膜上。

2）基底膜上面覆有单层扁平上皮，上面的上皮细胞特化增厚形成螺旋器。盖膜由螺旋缘伸出，覆盖在毛细胞上方。区分内、外毛细胞和支持细胞。

3）螺旋器中可见三角形的内隧道，支持细胞分内外两组排列在内隧道两旁。① 支持细胞：形态多样，可分为柱细胞和指细胞。柱细胞排列成两行，在内隧道的内侧为内柱细胞，外侧为外柱细胞。内、外柱细胞基部较宽，呈三角形，核圆形，细胞中部细长，互相分开，头部相连接，围成三角形的内隧道。指细胞也分内、外两组，内指细胞在内柱细胞的内侧，排成 1 排，外指细胞在外柱细胞外侧，排成 3～4 排，指细胞为柱状，核位于中部。② 毛细胞：分内毛细胞和外毛细胞，内毛细胞为 1 排，外毛细胞为 3～4 排，分别被内、外指细胞支托，每个毛细胞顶部有排列规则的静纤毛。盖膜是从螺旋缘伸出的一片胶质膜，生活状态下盖膜和静纤毛相接触，在切片中盖膜收缩与毛细胞脱离。

2.要求识别

（1）耳蜗。

（2）螺旋器。

二、复 习 思 考 题

（1）简述眼球壁的结构。

（2）简述角膜的结构特点。

（3）简述螺旋器的结构特点。

三、图片思考题

图 18 - 1   图 18 - 2

（陈　雪　程建青）

Chapter 18

EYE AND EAR

Learning Points

☞ The structure of the eyeball wall.

☞ The structural characteristics of the cornea and corneal limbus, the significance of scleral venous sinus, and the structures and functions of the iris, ciliary body and choroids.

☞ The structures and functions of the retina, and the structures and significances of the macula lutea and optic disc.

☞ The structures of osseous labyrinth and membranous labyrinth of the inner ear.

☞ The structures and functions of the crista ampullaris, maculae of saccule and utricle, and the structure and function of the spiral organ.

Part I   Experiment Contents

1. Eyeball wall

eyeball wall

A. Staining   HE.

(1) Low power:

1) The wall of the eyeball is composed of three layers: the outer tunica fibrosa, the intermediate tunica vasculosa, and the inner retina.

2) The pink stained cornea is located in the anterior 1/6 of the tunica fibrosa. The light red stained sclera forms the posterior 5/6.

3) The choroid lies beneath the sclera and contains large amount of pigment cells. Its forward extensions form ciliary body and iris.

4) Red stained lens lies behind the iris.

5) Occasional artificial retinal detachment is visible somewhere inside the choroid.

(2) High power:

1) Cornea: From the outside to the inside five sublayers can be distinguished as corneal epithelium, anterior limiting lamina, corneal stroma, posterior limiting lamina and corneal endothelium.

2) Sclera：It is a tough layer of dense connective tissue. The sclerocorneal junction, an area of transition from the the cornea to the the sclera, houses the $1\sim2$ lacunas, which are the scleral venous sinus lined by a thin layer of endothelium.

3) Iris：The anterior surface of the iris, i.e. the anterior border layer, is irregular and covered by a condensation of fibrocytes and melanocytes. The iris stroma consists of loose connective tissue rich in melanocytes and blood vessels. The posterior surface of the iris is covered by two layers of epithelium, and both are pigmented.

4) Ciliary body：It continues with iris. In transverse section, it is triangle in shape and contains short extensions, ciliary processes, towards the lens.

5) Choroid：It is located between the sclera and the retina and consists of loose connective tissue, which houses a dense network of blood vessel, and numerous melanocytes.

6) Retina：It is pressing against the inner surface of choroid, and retinal detachment from the choroid occurs only because of its contraction during the preparation of the slides. From the outside to the inside, the 10 sublayers of retina can be distinguished, of which four layers formed by nuclei are obvious：pigment epithelium, outer nuclear layer, inner nuclear layer and ganglion cells layer. The optic disc is the portion of the retina where the optic nerve leaves the eyeball. Since there are no photoreceptors, the visual field is blank and called as blind spot.

B. Identification requirements

（1）Cornea.

（2）Sclera.

（3）Ciliary body.

（4）Retina.

（5）Optic disc.

2. Inner ear

inner ear

A. Staining　　HE.

（1）Low power：

1) The cochlea, shaped like a snail-shell, is mainly formed by the bony structures.

2) The bony cone-shaped modiolus is located in the center of cochlea with two cross sections of the bony cochlear canal on both sides.

3) The spiral canal that forms the bony cochlea is divided into three distinct channels：an upper cavity, the scala vestibuli；a lower cavity, the scala tympani；and an intermediate cavity, the scala media （cochlear duct）. The scala vestibule is separated from the scala media by the vestibular membrane, whereas between the scala tympani and the scala media is the basilar membrane.

（2）High power：

1）The cochlear duct has the following histologic structure: Its upper wall is vestibular membrane which consists of two layers of squamous epithelium: one derivine from the scala media and the other from the lining of scala vestibuli. Its lateral wall is stria vascularis which is an unusual vascularized epithelium. The basal wall of cochlear duct is formed by the lateral portion of bony spiral lamina which is extended out from the modiolus and the basilar membrane, on which the spiral organ is located.

2）The upper surface of the basilar membrane is covered by a layer of simple squamous epithelium which differentidtes to form special receptor organ known as the spinal organ. Try to find inner and outer hair cells on the supporting cells. A gelatinous projection called tectorial membrane extends from the spiral limbus and sits on the top of hair cells.

3）Triangular section of inner tunnel is seen in the spiral organ, with the supporting cells standing on both sides of the inner tunnel. ① the supporting cells occur in 2 groups termed: the inner and outer pillar cells, and inner and outer phalangeal cells. The broad bases of the inner and outer pillar cells contain their nuclei, and their elongated upper part forming a triangular space between the outer and inner hair cells- the inner tunnel. The phalangeal cells also divide into 2 groups: the inner phalangeal cells are inside of the inner pillar cells, arranged in a row, and the outer phalangeal cells are outside of the outer pillar cells, arranged in 3 – 4 rows, underlie and support the sensory cells. ② the hair cells: There are two types of hair cells: inner hair cells, 1 row and outer hair cells, 3 – 4 row supporting by the inner and outer phalangeal cells respectively. These cells have stereocilia on free surface which are in contact with the tectorial membrane. The detachment is seen between the tectorial membrane and the hair cells because of the tectorial membrane contraction.

B. Identification requirements

（1）Cochlear duct.

（2）Spiral organ.

Part II　Questions for Review

（1）Briefly describe the structure of eyeball wall.

（2）Briefly describe the structural features of cornea.

（3）Briefly describe the structural features of spiral organ.

Part III　Pictures Questions for Review

Fig.18 – 1　　　　Fig.18 – 2

（Chen Xue，Cheng Jian Qing）

第十九章

人体胚胎发生总论

学习要点

☞ 两性生殖细胞的成熟,精子的获能。
☞ 受精、卵裂和胚泡形成及植入。
☞ 二胚层胚盘的形成及滋养层的分化。
☞ 三胚层胚盘的结构及其形成过程。
☞ 三胚层的分化及胚胎外形的建立。
☞ 胎膜与胎盘的结构和功能。

一、实 验 内 容

(一) 受精

观察受精的动画图片,并掌握受精的地点、过程及意义。

(二) 卵裂

卵裂在透明带内进行。卵裂模型一套有 4 个。透明带逐步溶解(第 1~4 天)。

1. 模型 1　　受精卵及三个极体。
2. 模型 2　　二细胞期。
3. 模型 3　　四细胞期。
4. 模型 4　　桑葚胚。

(三) 胚泡形成

模型 2　　胚泡(第 5 天,剖面观)

(1) 滋养层为胚泡腔周围的一层扁平细胞。

(2) 内细胞群是附在滋养层一侧的一团细胞。它向胚泡腔内突出,其附着处的滋养层称为极端滋养层。

(3) 胚泡腔:胚泡中央的一个大腔。

(四) 植入

植入模型一套有 4 个。植入后的子宫内膜称蜕膜。

1．模型 1　　（第 7 天）胚泡开始植入到子宫内膜中。

（1）极端滋养层细胞首先侵入子宫内膜。植入部位的滋养层开始分为两层：内层为细胞滋养层；外层为合体滋养层。

（2）内细胞群。

（3）胚泡腔。

2．模型 2　　（第 8 天）胚泡部分植入子宫内膜中。

（1）滋养层增殖，合体滋养层增多。

（2）由内细胞群分化出上胚层和下胚层，在上胚层的背侧出现羊膜腔。

3．模型 3　　（第 9 天）胚泡大部分植入子宫内膜中。

（1）滋养层继续增殖，合体滋养层内出现小腔隙。

（2）卵黄囊由下胚层边缘的细胞向下生长包围而成。

（3）上下胚层形成二胚层胚盘。

4．模型 4　　（第 12 天）胚泡全部植入子宫内膜内。

（1）滋养层继续发育，合体滋养层中腔隙增多并扩大。

（2）羊膜腔扩大。

（3）蜕膜分为三个部分：基蜕膜、包蜕膜、壁蜕膜。

（五）二胚层期（第 2 周）

此期的模型一套有 4 个。

1．模型 1

（1）滋养层：内层为细胞滋养层，外层为合体滋养层。

（2）胚泡腔。

（3）二胚层胚盘。

2．模型 2

（1）胚外中胚层：细胞滋养层向内分化形成。填充在细胞滋养层和卵黄囊之间。

（2）胚泡腔消失。

（3）二胚层胚盘。

3．模型 3

（1）合体滋养层范围扩大，内部出现许多小腔隙。

（2）胚外体腔：在胚外中胚层出现许多小腔融合成一个大腔形成。

（3）二胚层胚盘。

4．模型 4

（1）绒毛膜：由合体滋养层、细胞滋养层和胚外中胚层构成。在绒毛膜的表面有许多小突起称绒毛，分布均匀。

（2）胚外中胚层分为两层：位于卵黄囊外表面的称胚外脏壁中胚层；位于羊膜囊外面和细胞滋养层内面的称胚外体壁中胚层。

（3）体蒂：胚外中胚层在胚盘的尾端形成一条粗索称体蒂，是构成脐带的原基。

(六) 三胚层期(第 3 周)

此期的模型一套有 3 个。

1. 模型 1　　中胚层形成：在上胚层正中线的尾侧,部分上胚层细胞增生,形成一条纵行的细胞索称原条。原条的细胞在上、下胚层之间向周边扩展迁移,形成一个夹层,称中胚层(红色)。

2. 模型 2　　内胚层形成：原条的细胞进入下胚层,并逐渐置换下胚层的细胞,形成一层新的细胞,称内胚层(黄色)。

3. 模型 3　　外胚层形成：在内胚层和中胚层出现之后,原来上胚层改称外胚层(蓝色)。外、中、内三层构成三胚层胚盘。

(七) 胚体形成及胚层分化(第 3~8 周)

模型 1

(1) 胚体变成圆柱形：由于羊膜腔的扩大,三胚层胚盘向腹侧发生头褶、尾褶、左右侧褶；又由于中轴器官神经系统和体节的形成,胚体向背部突出,整个胚体呈圆柱形。

(2) 神经管的形成：神经板→ 神经沟→ 神经褶→ 神经管(含前、后神经孔)前神经孔愈合形成脑；后神经孔愈合形成脊髓。

(3) 中胚层分为三部分：① 轴旁中胚层：形成体节。② 间介中胚层。③ 侧中胚层：出现胚内体腔,分为体壁中胚层和脏壁中胚层。

(4) 原始消化管的形成：在胚体形成的同时,内胚层卷褶形成原始消化管。其分为三段：① 前肠：包在头褶内的部分,有口咽膜封口。② 中肠：与卵黄囊相连的一段。③ 后肠：包在尾褶内的部分,有泄殖腔膜封堵。

(八) 胎膜与胎盘

1. 观察模型　　胎儿、胎膜、胎盘与子宫的关系。
2. 蜕膜　　分为三部分：① 包蜕膜；② 壁蜕膜；③ 基蜕膜。
3. 胎膜　　包括绒毛膜、羊膜、卵黄囊、尿囊和脐带。

(1) 绒毛膜：由滋养层和胚外中胚层组成。发育为平滑绒毛膜和丛密绒毛膜。

(2) 羊膜：由羊膜上皮和胚外中胚层组成。

(3) 卵黄囊：大部分退化成细长的卵黄蒂,被包于脐带中,最后消失。

(4) 尿囊：为细长的盲管,被包于脐带中,最后消失。

(5) 脐带：以体蒂为基础,外包有羊膜,内含卵黄囊、尿囊和脐带血管。

4. 胎盘　　由胎儿的丛密绒毛膜和母体的基蜕膜组成。

二、复 习 思 考 题

(1) 简述受精的时间、地点和过程及受精的意义。

(2) 简述植入的定义、时间及过程。

(3) 简述三胚层的分化。

(4) 简述胎膜的构成及演变。

（5）简述胎盘的形成、结构及功能。

三、图 片 复 习 题

图 19-1　　　　　　　　图 19-2　　　　　　　　图 19-3

（陈永珍　张于娟）

Chapter 19

GENERAL HUMAN EMBRYOLOGY

Learning Points

☞ Mature of germ cells in the male and female, and sperm capacitation.
☞ Fertilization, cleavage, blastocyst formation and implantation.
☞ Formation of the bilaminar germ disc and trophoblast differentiation.
☞ Structure and formation of the trilaminar germ disc.
☞ Differentiation of three germ layers and establishment of the shape of the embryo.
☞ Structure and function of the fetal membrane and placenta.

Part I   Experiment Contents

1. Fertilization

Observe the animated cartoon of the fertilization, and focus on its site, whole process and significance.

2. Cleavage

Cleavage takes place inside the zona pellucida. There are 4 models (one set) to show the cleavage, the zona pellucida dissoved gradually (day 1 to 4).

A. Model 1   Fertilized ovum and three polar bodies.
B. Model 2   Two cell stage.
C. Model 3   Four cell stage.
D. Model 4   Morula.

3. Blastocyst formation

Model 2   Blastocyst (day 5, profile view)

(1) The trophoblast is a layer of flat cells surrounding the blastocyst cavity.

(2) The inner cell mass is a group of centrally located cells, which projects into the blastocyst cavity. The trophoblast that the inner cell mass attached is called polar trophoblast.

(3) The blastocyst cavity is a central cavity of the blastocyst.

4. Implantation

There are 4 models (1 set) to show implantation. After implantation the endometrium is named the decidua.

A. Model 1   The blastocyst begins to implant into endometrium (day 7).

(1) The polar trophoblast cells first invade the endometrium and begin to divide into two layers: the inner cytotrophoblast and outer syncytiotrophoblast.

(2) The inner cell mass.

(3) The blastocyst cavity.

B. Model 2   The blastocyst partly implants into the endometrium (day 8).

(1) The trophoblast proliferates and the amount of syncytiotrophoblast increases.

(2) The inner cell mass differentiates to form the epiblast and hypoblast, and the amniotic cavity appears on the dorsal surface of the epiblast.

C. Model 3   Most part of the blastocyst implants into the endometrium (day 9).

(1) The trophoblast continues to proliferate and small lacunae appear in the syncytiotrophoblast.

(2) Yolk sac is formed by the cells of the edge of the hypoblast which proliferate and migrate out over cytotrophoblast.

(3) Bilaminar embryonic disc is well formed.

D. Model 4   The blastocyst implants into endometrium completely (day 12).

(1) The trophoblast continues to develop and the lacunae in syncytiotrophoblast expand and increase in numbers.

(2) The amniotic cavity expands.

(3) The decidua is divided into three parts: decidua basalis, decidua capsularis and decidua parietalis.

5. Bilaminar Germ Disc (2nd week)

There are 4 models (1 set).

A. Model 1

(1) The trophoblast is divided into layers: inner cytotrophoblast and outer syncytiotrophoblast.

(2) The blastocyst cavity.

(3) The bilaminar germ disc.

B. Model 2

(1) The extraembryonic mesoderm arises from the inner surface of the cytotrophoblast, and its cells fill the space between yolk sac and cytotrophoblast.

(2) The blastocyst cavity disappears.

(3) The bilaminar germ disc.

C. Model 3

(1) The syncytiotrophoblast expands and many small lacunae appear inside.

(2) The extraembryonic coelom is formed by many small cavities in the extraembryonic mesoderm which fuse into a large cavity.

(3) The bilaminar germ disc.

D. Model 4

(1) The chorion is composed of cytotrophoblast, syncytiotrophoblast and extraembryonic mesoderm, and many evenly distributed small processes on its surface are called villi.

(2) The extraembryonic mesoderm is divided into two layers: extraembryonic splanchnopleuric mesoderm which lies on the outer surface of yolk sac, and extraembryonic somatopleuric mesoderm which lies on the outer surface of amnion and the inner surface of the cytotrophoblast.

(3) The connecting (body) stalk is a thick rope at the end of the embryonic disc formed by extraembryonic mesoderm, which constitutes the umbilical cord primordium.

6. Trilaminar germ disc (3rd week)

There are 3 models (one set).

A. Model 1   Formation of mesoderm: Cells of the epiblast first forms primitive streak, and then the cells of primitive streak extend further between epiblast and hypoblast forming intraembryonic mesoderm (red layer).

B. Model 2   Formation of endoderm: Primitive streak cells migrate into the hypoblast and gradually replaces the hypoblast cells forming a new layer of cells called the endoderm (yellow layer).

C. Model 3   Formation of ectoderm: Once endoderm and mesoderm appear, the original epiblast is renamed ectoderm (blue layer), then the endoderm, mesoderm and ectoderm constitute the trilaminar germ disc.

7. Differentiation of germ layers and establishment of body form (3rd to 8th week)

Model 1

(1) Cylindrical embryo: As the result of amniotic cavity expansion, rapid growth of central nervous system, somites, and the folding of the embryo produce the head, tail and lateral folds, making the embryo looks like a cylinder.

(2) The formation of the neural tube: The neural plate rapidly elongates and broadens, and then invaginates along its central axis to form a neural groove and neural folds on each side. The neural folds fuse along their length to form the neural tube which forms all the components of brain and spinal cord.

(3) The mesoderm is divided into 3 parts: ① paraxial mesoderm which forms somite, ② intermediate mesoderm, and ③ lateral mesoderm which is composed of extraembryonic splanchnopleuric mesoderm and extraembryonic somatopleuric mesoderm.

（4）The formation of the primitive digestive tract: As the flat embryonic disc itself folds into a somewhat cylindrical embryo, the primitive gut is formed by the endoderm and divided into three segment: ① Foregut, the part enclosed in the head fold and sealed by oropharyngeal membrane; ② midgut connects with yolksac; ③ hindgut, the part enclosed in caudal fold.

8. Fetal membranes and placenta

（1）Observe the relationship of the fetus, fetal membranes, placenta and uterus.

（2）The decidua is divided into 3 parts: ① decidua basalis; ② decidua capsularis; ③ decidua parietalis.

（3）Fetal membranes include chorion, amnion, yolk sac, allantois and umbilical cord.

1）The chorion is composed of syncytiotrophoblast, cytotrophobalst and extraembryonic mesoderm within villi, and develops into two types, chorion frondosum and chorion leave.

2）The amnion is a thin, transparent membrane formed by amniotic cell layer and outer extraembryonic mesoderm layer.

3）The yolk sac mostly degenerates into a slender yolk pedicle, and is wrapped in the umbilical cord.

4）The allantois is a finger-like diverticulum from the caudal part of the yolk sac, extending into body stalk.

5）Based on the body pedicle, the umbilical is covered with amniotic membrane and contains the structures of yolk sac, allantois and umbilical vessels.

（4）The placenta consists of two components: fetal component developing from chorion frondosum, and maternal component developing from decidua basalis.

Part II   Questions for Review

（1）Briefly describe the time, site, process and significance of the fertilization.
（2）Briefly describe the definition, time and process of implantation.
（3）Briefly describe the differentiation of the three germ layers.
（4）Briefly describe the composition and evolution of the fetal membranes.
（5）Briefly describe the formation, structure and function of the placenta.

Part III   Pictures Questions for Review

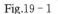

Fig.19 - 1   Fig.19 - 2   Fig.19 - 3

（Chen Yongzhen, Zhang Yujuan）

第二十章

颜面和腭的发生

学习要点

☞ 鳃弓、鳃沟的发生。

☞ 颜面的发生。

☞ 腭的发生。

☞ 颜面发生中常见的先天性畸形。

一、实 验 内 容

（一）鳃弓的发生

模型　第4周胚胎头部。

（1）额鼻突。

（2）眼泡。

（3）鳃弓。

（4）鳃沟。

（二）颜面的形成

1. 模型1

（1）第一鳃弓腹侧分上下两支,形成上颌突和下颌突。

（2）颜面有五个突起即是：额鼻突,一对上颌突和一对下颌突。

（3）五个突起围成的中央凹陷称为口凹。

（4）额鼻突下缘两侧有一对鼻窝。

2. 模型2

（1）外侧鼻突形成。

（2）内侧鼻突形成。

3. 模型3

（1）上颌突与同侧外侧鼻突融合形成鼻泪沟。

（2）上颌突与同侧内侧鼻突融合形成上唇外侧部分与上颌。

（3）左右内侧鼻突在中线融合形成上唇正中部分和人中。

（4）左右下颌突在中线融合形成下颌和下唇。

二、复习思考题

(1) 颜面的原基是什么？

(2) 简述颜面的常见畸形。

三、图片复习题

图 20-1

图 20-2

（李　奕）

Chapter 20

THE DEVELOPMENT OF FACE AND PALATE

Learning Points

☞ The development of branchial arch and branchial grooves.
☞ The development of the face.
☞ The development of the palate.
☞ Common congenital malformations in the development of face.

Part I   Experiment Contents

1. The development of branchial arch

Model   The head of 4 week embryo.
(1) Frontonasal prominence.
(2) Optic vesicle.
(3) Branchial arch.
(4) Branchial groove.

2. The formation of face

A. Model 1

(1) The ventral side of the first branchial arch is divided into two branches, forming a maxillary prominence and a mandibular prominence.

(2) The face has five prominence: frontonasal prominence, a pair of maxillary prominences and a pair of mandibular prominences.

(3) The five prominences form a central depression called the stomodeum.

(4) A pair of nasal fossae rest on the lower edge of the frontonasal prominence on both sides.

B. Model 2

(1) Formation of lateral nasal prominence.

（2）Formation of medial nasal prominence.

C. Model 3

（1）The maxillary prominence merges with ipsilateral lateral nasal prominence to form nasolacrimal groove.

（2）The maxillary prominence merges with ipsilateral medial nasal prominence to form upper jaw and laleral upper lip.

（3）Left and right medial nasal prominences merge in the midline to form the middle part of the upper lip and philtrum.

（4）The left and right mandibular prominence merge in the midline to form the lower jaw and lip.

Part II　Questions for Review

（1）What are the primordia of the face?

（2）Briefly describe briefly the congenital malformations of the face.

Part III　Pictures Questions for Review

Fig.20 - 1　　　　Fig.20 - 2

（Li Yi）

第二十一章

消化系统与呼吸系统的发生

学习要点

☞ 咽囊的演变。

☞ 原始消化管的形成与分化。

☞ 甲状腺的发生及常见的先天性畸形。

☞ 消化管、肝和胰的发生及常见的先天性畸形。

☞ 气管和肺的发生及常见的先天性畸形。

一、实 验 内 容

(一) 咽囊的演变及甲状腺的发生

模型　　原始咽。

(1) 第 1 对咽囊分化为中耳鼓室和咽鼓管。

(2) 第 2 对咽囊分化腭扁桃体上皮和隐窝。

(3) 第 3 对咽囊腹侧分化形成胸腺,背侧分化形成下一对甲状旁腺。

(4) 第 4 对咽囊背侧分化形成上一对甲状旁腺。

(5) 第 5 对咽囊分化形成后鳃体。

(6) 甲状舌管由原始咽的底部形成,其末端分化为甲状腺。

(二) 原始消化管的演变

模型　　原始消化管分为前肠、中肠和后肠。

(1) 前肠的演变

1) 5 对咽囊。

2) 甲状腺原基。

3) 喉气管憩室。

4) 食管。

5) 胃。

6) 十二指肠上段。

7) 肝、胆囊。

8) 腹胰、背胰。

（2）中肠的演变

1）中肠袢形成。

2）卵黄蒂出现最后消失。

3）中肠袢的旋转。

4）中肠演变为十二指肠下段至空肠，回肠，升结肠和横结肠右 2/3。

（3）后肠的演变

1）后肠末端膨大称泄殖腔。

2）泄殖腔分隔形成尿生殖窦和原始直肠。

3）后肠演变为横结肠左 1/3 至降结肠，乙状结肠，直肠和肛管上段。

（三）呼吸系统的发生

（1）喉气管沟的形成。

（2）喉气管沟加深延伸形成喉气管憩室，其末端膨大称肺芽。

（3）肺芽是支气管和肺的原基。

二、复习思考题

（1）简述前、中、后肠的演变。

（2）肝脏、胰腺以及呼吸系统的原基是什么？

（3）简述泄殖腔的分隔过程及相关的常见先天性畸形。

（4）简述消化、呼吸系统常见的先天性畸形。

三、图片复习题

图 21-1　　　　　　图 21-2

（吴　坚）

Chapter 21

THE DEVELOPMENT OF THE DIGESTIVE AND RESPRATORY SYSTEMS

Learning Points

☞ The derivatives of the pharyngeal pouches.

☞ The formation and differentiation of the primitive gut.

☞ The development and common congenital malformations of the thyroid gland.

☞ The development and common congenital malformations of the digestive tract, the liver and the pancreas.

☞ The development and common congenital malformations of the trachea and the lung.

Part I Experiment Contents

1. The evolution of the pharyngeal pouches and the development of the thyroid

Model   Primitive pharynx.

(1) The 1st pair of pharyngeal pouches differentiate into the tympanums of the middle ear and the eustachian tube.

(2) The 2nd pair of pharyngeal pouches differentiate into the palatine tonsil epithelium and crypts.

(3) The 3rd pair of pharyngeal pouches expand to form ventral and dorsal portions, the ventral portions differentiate into the thymus and the dorsal portions differentiate into the lower pair of the parathyroid glands.

(4) The dorsal portions of the 4th pair of pharyngeal pouches differentiate into the upper pair of the parathyroid glands.

(5) The 5th pair of the pharyngeal pouches differentiate into the ultimobranchial body.

(6) The thyroglossal duct is formed by the floor of the primitive pharynx and its

terminal portion differentiates into the thyroid.

2. The evolution of the primitive gut

Model   The primitive gut is divided into the foregut, the midgut and the hindgut.

(1) The evolution of the foregut

1) Five pairs of the pharyngeal pouches.

2) The thyroid primordium.

3) The laryngotracheal diverticulum.

4) The esophagus.

5) The stomach.

6) The duodenum upper segment.

7) The liver and cholecyst.

8) The ventral pancreas and the dorsal pancreas.

(2) The evolution of the midgut

1) The formation of the midgut loop.

2) The appearance of the yolk stalk.

3) Rotation of the midgut loop.

4) The midgut evolves into the lower segment of the duodenum, jejunum, ileum, ascending colon and the right two thirds of the transverse colon.

(3) The evolution of the hindgut

1) The terminal enlargement of the hindgut forms the cloaca.

2) The cloaca is divided into the urogenital sinus and the primitive rectum.

3) The hindgut evolves into the left one third of the transverse colon, descending colon, sigmoid colon, rectum and the upper segment of the anal canal.

3. The development of the respiratory system

(1) The formation of the laryngotracheal groove.

(2) The laryngotracheal groove deepens and extends to form the laryngotracheal diverticulum, whose terminal enlargement is called the lung bud.

(3) The lung bud is the primordia of the bronchi and the lung.

Part II   Questions for Review

(1) Briefly describe the derivatives of the foregut, midgut and hindgut.

(2) What are the primordia of the liver, the pancreas, and the respiratory system?

(3) Briefly describe the procedure for the partitioning of the cloaca, and related common congenital malformations.

(4) Briefly describe the common congenital malformations of the digestive and respiratory systems.

Part III   Pictures Questions for Review

Fig.21 - 1

Fig.21 - 2

(Wu Jian)

第二十二章

泌尿系统与生殖系统的发生

学习要点

☞ 中肾小管及中肾管的发生。
☞ 后肾的发生。
☞ 泄殖腔的分隔及演变。
☞ 泌尿系统常见的畸形。
☞ 生殖腺及生殖管道的发生。
☞ 生殖系统常见的畸形。

一、实 验 内 容

(一) 泌尿系统的发生

模型　　胚胎躯体尾端的横断面。
(1) 尿生殖嵴外侧隆起为中肾嵴,内侧隆起为生殖腺嵴。
(2) 尿直肠隔自头端向尾端分隔泄殖腔。分隔后,腹侧为尿生殖窦,背侧为原始直肠。
(3) 后肾沿胚胎背侧体壁向头端迁移。
(4) 中肾管通入泄殖腔。
(5) 泄殖腔腹侧通尿囊,背侧上方通后肠。

(二) 生殖系统的发生

模型　　胚胎腹后部两侧的表面观。
(1) 尿生殖嵴内侧的隆起为生殖腺嵴,内有睾丸或卵巢发生。
(2) 尿生殖嵴外侧的隆起为中肾嵴,内有中肾。
(3) 中肾管和中肾旁管,是生殖管道分化的原基。

二、复 习 思 考 题

(1) 简述前肾、中肾和后肾的形成和归宿。
(2) 简述泌尿系统的常见畸形及其形成原因。
(3) 简述生殖腺的原基及睾丸和卵巢的发生。

（4）简述性未分化期，男女两性同时具有的两套生殖管道和它们的归宿。

（5）简述尿生殖窦的演变。

三、图 片 思 考 题

图 22 - 1

图 22 - 2

（林巍巍）

Chapter 22

THE DEVELOPMENT OF THE URINARY AND REPRODUCTIVE SYSTEMS

Learning Points

☞ The development of mesonephric tubule and mesonephric duct.

☞ The development of metanephros.

☞ The partitioning and evolution of cloaca.

☞ The common malformations of the urinary system.

☞ The development of gonads and genital ducts.

☞ The common malformations of the reproductive system.

Part I   Experiment Contents

1. The development of the urinary system

Model   Cross-section of the caudal portion of the embryo.

(1) The lateral portion of the urogenital ridge bulges to form the mesonephric ridge and the medial portion bulges to form the gonadal ridge.

(2) Urorectal septum separates the cloaca from the cranial end to the caudal end. After the separation, the ventral portion is named the urogenital sinus and the dorsal protion is named the anorectal canal.

(3) The metanephros is migrating to the cranial part of the dorsal surface of the embryonic coelom (body cavity).

(4) The mesonephric tube is connected with the cloaca laterally.

(5) The ventral portion of cloaca is connected with the allantois, and the dorsal portion is connected with the hindgut.

2. The development of the reproductive system

Model   Surface view of both sides of the abdomen.

（1）The medial portion urogenital ridge bulges to form the gonadal ridge，where the testis or the ovary develope.

（2）The lateral portion urogenital ridge bulges to form the mesonephric ridge，where the mesonephridium develope.

（3）The mesonephric duct and the paramesonephric duct are the primordia of reproductive tract.

Part II　Questions for Review

（1）Briefly describe the formation and the fate of the pronephros, mesonephros, and metanephros.

（2）Briefly describe the common congenital malformations of the urinary system and how are they formed.

（3）Briefly describe the primordium of the gonad and how do the testis and the ovary develop respectively.

（4）At the undifferentiated stage of sex, both male and female embryos have two pairs of genital ducts. Briefly describe what are they and what are their fates.

（5）Briefly describe the evolution of the urogenital sinus.

Part III　Pictures Questions for Review

Fig.22 - 1　　　　　Fig.22 - 2

（Lin Weiwei）

第二十三章

心血管系统的发生

学习要点

☞ 血岛的发生与早期血循环的建立。
☞ 心管的形成和位置变化,心脏外形的演变和内部分隔。
☞ 心血管系统的常见畸形。
☞ 胎儿血循环的途径、特点及其出生后的变化。

一、实 验 内 容

(一) 心脏外形的演变

模型

(1) 心管由心球、心室、心房和静脉窦组成,呈"S"形弯曲。
(2) 心球心室形成球室袢并凸向腹、尾、右侧。
(3) 心房移向背、头侧,并向心球两侧扩张。
(4) 心球尾端形成原始右心室,原心室形成原始左心室。

(二) 心脏内部的分隔

模型

(1) 第一房间隔出现,其尾侧缘下方有第一房间孔。
(2) 第一房间孔封闭,同时在第一房间隔上部形成第二房间孔。
(3) 第二房间隔形成,并覆盖第二房间孔,其尾侧缘下方有卵圆孔。
(4) 第一房间隔的留存部分形成卵圆孔瓣。
(5) 心室内室间隔肌部已形成,室间孔被室间隔膜部完全封闭。

二、复 习 思 考 题

(1) 简述心管的形成与分部。
(2) 简述原始心房、原始心室的分隔。
(3) 简述胎儿血液循环的特点以及出生后的变化。
(4) 简述心血管系统常见畸形及其形成机制。
(5) 简述房间隔缺损与空间隔缺损的形成原因。

（6）简述法洛四联症的形成原因和症状。

三、图片思考题

图 23-1

图 23-2

图 23-3

（姚　健）

Chapter 23

THE DEVELOPMENT OF THE CARDIOVASCULAR SYSTEM

Learning Points

☞ The development of blood island and the establishment of early blood circulation.
☞ The formation and positional changes of the heart tube, and the evolution of the external appearance and the internal septation of the heart.
☞ Common malformations of the cardiovascular system.
☞ The pathway, characteristics of fetal blood circulation and its changes after birth.

Part I   Experiment Contents

1. Evolution of the external appearance of the heart

Model

(1) The cardiac tube curved in the shape of "S" is formed by bulbus cordis, ventricle, atrium and sinus venosus.

(2) The bulboventricular portion grows faster and forms bulboventricular loop which bends ventrally, caudally and slightly to the right.

(3) The atrium moves dorsocranially and bulges laterally on each side of bulbus cordis.

(4) The proximal part of bulbus cordis forms the primitive right ventricle, while original ventricle forms the primitive left ventricle.

2. Internal septation of the heart

Model

(1) The septum primum is well formed with foramen primum below its caudal free edge.

(2) As the upper part of septum primum is absorbed, the foramen secundum is

formed on top and the foramen primum is closed.

(3) The septum secundum is formed covering the foramen secundum and leaves the foramen ovale below its lower edge.

(4) The remaining portion of septum primum forms the valve of the oval foramen.

(5) The muscular part of interventricular septum is formed, and the interventricular foramen is completely closed by the membranous part of the interventricular septum.

Part II　Questions for Review

(1) Briefly describe the formation and subdivisions of the heart tube.

(2) Briefly describe the internal septation of the primitive atrium and ventricle.

(3) Briefly describe the characteristics of fetal circulation and its changes after birth.

(4) Briefly describe the common congenital malformations of the cardiovascular system and the related mechanisms.

(5) Briefly describe the causes of the atrial septal defect and the ventricular septal defect.

(6) Briefly describe the causes and the symptoms of the tetralogy of Fallot.

Part III　Pictures Questions for Review

Fig.23 - 1

Fig.23 - 2

Fig.23 - 3

(Yao Jian)

图片思考题
答案

附 录

词汇表 Glossary

上 皮 组 织

glossary epithelial tissue　上皮组织

covering epithelium　被覆上皮

pseudostratified ciliated columnar epithelium
　假复层纤毛柱状上皮

endothelium　内皮

mesothelium　间皮

simple squamous epithelium　单层扁平上皮

simple cuboidal epithelium　单层立方上皮

simple columnar epithelium　单层柱状上皮

stratified squamous epithelium　复层扁平上皮

striated border　纹状缘

transitional epithelium　变移上皮

cell coat　细胞衣

microvillus　微绒毛

cilium　纤毛

tight junction　紧密连接

intermediate junction　中间连接

desmosome　桥粒

gap junction　缝隙连接

basement membrane　基膜

plasma membrane infolding　质膜内褶

hemidesmosome　半桥粒

固有结缔组织

connective tissue　结缔组织

connective tissue proper　固有结缔组织

loose connective tissue　疏松结缔组织

dense connective tissue　致密结缔组织

reticular tissue　网状组织

adipose tissue　脂肪组织

fibroblast　成纤维细胞

macrophage　巨噬细胞

plasma cell　浆细胞

mast cell　肥大细胞

fat cell　脂肪细胞

fibroblast　成纤维细胞

fibrocyte　纤维细胞

ground substance　基质

collagenous fiber　胶原纤维

elastic fiber　弹性纤维

reticular fiber　网状纤维

reticular cell　网状细胞

reticular tissue　网状组织

血　　液

blood　血液

serum　血清

blood plasma　血浆

Wright's staining　瑞氏染色

hemocyte　血细胞

erythrocyte　红细胞

hemoglobin(Hb)　血红蛋白

reticulocyte　网织红细胞

leukocyte　白细胞

granulocyte　有粒白细胞

agranulocyte　无粒白细胞

azurophilic granule　嗜天青颗粒

neutrophil（neutrophilic granulocyte）　中性粒
　细胞

eosinophil　嗜酸性粒细胞

basophil　嗜碱性粒细胞

monocyte　单核细胞

lymphocyte　淋巴细胞

blood platelet　血小板

软 骨 和 骨

cartilage　软骨

cartilage tissue　软骨组织

hyaline cartilage　透明软骨

elastic cartilage　弹性软骨

fibrous cartilage/fibrocartilage　纤维软骨

chondrocyte　软骨细胞

isogenous group　同源细胞群

perichondrium　软骨膜

cartilage lacuna　软骨陷窝

cartilage capsule　软骨囊

hyaline cartilage　透明软骨

bone　骨

osseous tissue/bone tissue　骨组织

bone matrix　骨质

osteoprogenitor cell　骨祖细胞

osteoblast　成骨细胞

osteocyte　骨细胞

osteoclast　破骨细胞

circumferential lamella　环骨板

osteon　骨单位

osteoprogenitor cell　骨原细胞

Haversian system　哈弗斯系统

Haversian canal　哈弗斯管

Haversian lamella　哈弗斯骨板

interstitial lamella　间骨板

periosteum　骨外膜

endosteum　骨内膜

肌 组 织

muscle tissue　　肌组织

muscle fiber　肌纤维

sarcolemma　肌膜

sarcoplasm　肌浆

sarcoplasmic reticulum　肌浆网

skeletal muscle　骨骼肌

epimysium　肌外膜

perimysium　肌束膜

endomysium　肌内膜

striated muscle　横纹肌

myofilament　肌丝

isotropic band　I 带

anisotropic band　A 带

light band　明带

dark band　暗带

sarcomere　肌节

myofibril　肌原纤维

transverse tubule（T tubule）　横小管

longitudinal tubule　纵小管

terminal cisterna　终池

triad　三联体

cardiac muscle　心肌

intercalated disc　闰盘

diad　二联体

smooth muscle　平滑肌

神 经 组 织

nervous tissue　神经组织

nerve cell　神经细胞

neuroglial cell　神经胶质细胞

neuron　神经元

soma　胞体

axon　突起

dendrite　树突

axon　轴突

axon hillock　轴丘

Nissl body　尼氏体

neurofibril　神经原纤维

neurofilament　神经丝

microtubule　微管

synapse　突触

chemical synapse　化学性突触

presynaptic element　突触前成分

synaptic vesicle　突触小泡

synaptic cleft　突触间隙

postsynaptic element　突触后成分

glial cell　胶质细胞

gray matter　灰质

white matter　白质

astrocyte　星形胶质细胞

oligodendrocyte　少突胶质细胞

microglia　小胶质细胞

ependyma　室管膜

ependymal cell 室管膜细胞

Schwann cell 施万细胞

neurilemmal cell 神经膜细胞

satellite cell 卫星细胞

nerve fiber 神经纤维

myelinated nerve fiber 有髓神经纤维

unmyelinated nerve fiber 无髓神经纤维

mesaxon 轴突系膜

myelin sheath 髓鞘

neurilemma 神经膜

Ranvier node 郎飞结

internode 结间体

nerve 神经

epineurium 神经外膜

perineurium 神经束膜

endoneurium 神经内膜

sensory nerve ending 感觉神经末梢

free nerve ending 游离神经末梢

encapsulated nerve ending 被囊神经末梢

tactile corpuscle 触觉小体

lamellar corpuscle 环层小体

muscle spindle 肌梭

motor nerve ending 运动神经末梢

somatic motor nerve ending 躯体运动神经末梢

visceral motor nerve ending 内脏运动神经末梢

motor end plate 运动终板

循 环 系 统

circulatory system 循环系统

cardiovascular system 心血管系统

heart 心

walls of heart 心脏壁层

endocardium 心内膜

endothelium 内皮

subendothelial layer 内皮下层

subendocardial layer 心内膜下层

Purkinje fibers 浦肯野纤维

myocardium 心肌膜

epicardium 心外膜

pacemaker cell 起搏细胞

artery 动脉

medium-sized artery 中动脉

muscular artery 肌性动脉

tunica intima 内膜

internal elastic membrane 内弹性膜

tunica media 中膜

tunica adventitia 外膜

external elastic membrane 外弹性膜

large artery 大动脉

elastic artery 弹性动脉

small artery 小动脉

arteriole 微动脉

capillary 毛细血管

continuous capillary 连续性毛细血管

fenestrated capillary 有孔毛细血管

discontinuous sinusoidal capillary 不连续毛细血管

blood sinusoid 血窦

sinusoid capillary 窦状毛细血管

vein 静脉

venule 微静脉

免 疫 系 统

immune System 免疫系统

lymphatic system 淋巴系统

lymphatic capillary 毛细淋巴管

lymphatic trunks 淋巴干

lymphatic ducts 淋巴导管

lymphoid organ 淋巴器官

central lymphoid organ 中枢淋巴器官

peripheral lymphoid organ 周围淋巴器官

lymphatic tissue 淋巴组织

diffuse lymphoid tissue 弥散淋巴组织

lymphoid nodule 淋巴小结

immune cell 免疫细胞

germinal center 生发中心

high endothelial venule 高内皮微静脉

T cell T 细胞

B cell B 细胞

thymus 胸腺

capsule 被膜

interlobular septum 小叶间隔

thymocyte 胸腺细胞

thymic epithelial cell 胸腺上皮细胞

thymic corpuscle 胸腺小体

lymphoid node 淋巴结

trabecula　小梁

cortical sinus　皮质淋巴窦

subcapsular sinus　被膜下淋巴窦

peritrabecular sinus　小梁周窦

superficial cortex　浅层皮质

paracortex zone　副皮质区

thymus dependent area　胸腺依赖区

medullary cord　髓索

medullary sinus　髓窦

spleen　脾

white pulp　白髓

periarterial lymphatic sheath　动脉周围淋巴鞘

central artery　中央动脉

splenic corpuscle　脾小结

red pulp　红髓

splenic cord　脾索

splenic sinus　脾窦

marginal zone　边缘区

palatine tonsil　腭扁桃体

消 化 系 统

digestive system　消化系统

digestive tract　消化管

mucosa　黏膜

lamina propria　固有层

muscularis mucosa　黏膜肌层

submucosa　黏膜下层

muscularis　肌层

adventitia　外膜

tongue　舌

lingual papilla　舌乳头

filiform papilla　丝状乳头

fungiform papilla　菌状乳头

circumvallate papilla　轮廓乳头

esophagus　食管

esophageal gland　食管腺

stomach　胃

fundic gland　胃底腺

chief cell　主细胞

zymogen cell　胃酶细胞

parietal cell　壁细胞

oxyntic cell　泌酸细胞

mucous neck cell　颈黏液细胞

small intestine　小肠

plica circularis　环行皱襞

absorptive cell　吸收细胞

striated border　纹状缘

goblet cell　杯状细胞

endocrine cell　内分泌细胞

small intestinal gland　小肠腺

Paneth cell　帕内特细胞

undifferentiated cell　未分化细胞

intestinal villus　肠绒毛

large intestine　大肠

Peyer's patch；aggregated lymphoid nodules　派
　尔集合淋巴结

消 化 腺

digestive gland　消化腺

pancreas　胰腺

acinus　腺泡

exocrine portion　外分泌部

pancreas islet　胰岛

centroacinar cell　泡心细胞

intercalated duct　闰管

glucagon　高血糖素

insulin　胰岛素

somatostatin　生长抑素

liver　肝

hepatic lobule/liver lobule　肝小叶

hepatic plate/liver plate　肝板

limiting plate　界板

hepatocyte　肝细胞

Kupffer cell　库普弗细胞

hepatic sinusoid　肝血窦

Disse space　狄氏间隙

perisinusoidal space　窦周隙

bile canaliculus　胆小管

portal area　门管区

interlobular vein　小叶间静脉

interlobular artery　小叶间动脉

interlobular bile duct　小叶间胆管

呼 吸 系 统

respiratory system　呼吸系统

trachea　气管

lung　肺

conducting portion　导气部

lobar bronchus　叶支气管

small bronchus　小支气管

bronchiole　细支气管

terminal bronchiole　终末细支气管

respiratory portion　呼吸部

respiratory bronchiole　呼吸性细支气管

alveolar duct　肺泡管

alveolar sac　肺泡囊

pulmonary alveolus　肺泡

alveolar epithelium　肺泡上皮

type Ⅰ alveolar cell　Ⅰ型肺泡细胞

type Ⅱ alveolar cell　Ⅱ型肺泡细胞

surfactant　表面活性物质

alveolar septum　肺泡隔

alveolar pore　肺泡孔

pulmonary macrophage　肺巨噬细胞

dust cell　尘细胞

supporting cell　支持细胞

blood-air barrier　血-气屏障

respiratory membrane　呼吸膜

泌 尿 系 统

urinary system　泌尿系统

kidney　肾

renal cortex　肾皮质

renal medulla　肾髓质

cortical labyrinth　皮质迷路

medullary ray　髓放线

uriniferous tubule　泌尿小管

nephron　肾单位

vascular pole　血管极

urinary pole　尿极

renal corpuscle　肾小体

glomerulus　血管球（肾小球）

mesangium　血管系膜

mesangial cell　系膜细胞

mesangial matrix　系膜基质

renal capsule　肾小囊

parietal layer　壁层

visceral layer　脏层

capsular space　肾小囊腔

podocyte　足细胞

slit membrane　裂孔膜

filtration membrane　滤过膜

filtration barrier　滤过屏障

renal tubule　肾小管

proximal tubule　近端小管

thin segment　细段

distal tubule　远端小管

pars convoluta　曲部

pars recta　直部

proximal convoluted tubule　近曲小管

brush border　刷状缘

lateral process　侧突

basal striation　基底纵纹

distal convoluted tubule　远曲小管

collection tubule　集合管

juxtaglomerular complex　球旁复合体

juxtaglomerular apparatus　肾小球旁器

juxtaglomerular cell　球旁细胞

renin　肾素

macula densa　致密斑

extraglomerular mesangial cell　球外系膜细胞

内 分 泌 系 统

endocrine system　内分泌系统

endocrine gland　内分泌腺

nitrogen-containing hormone secretory cell　含氮激素分泌细胞

steroid hormone secretory cell　类固醇激素分泌细胞

thyroid gland　甲状腺

thyroid hormone　甲状腺激素

follicular epithelial cell　滤泡上皮细胞

iodinated thyroglobulin　碘化的甲状腺球蛋白

colloid　胶体

thyroxine　甲状腺素

triiodothyronine(T3)　三碘甲状腺原氨酸

tetraiodothyronine(T4)　四碘甲状腺原氨酸

parafollicular cell　滤泡旁细胞

calcitonin　降钙素

parathyroid gland　甲状旁腺

chief cell　主细胞

parathyroid hormone　甲状旁腺激素

oxyphil cell　嗜酸性细胞

adrenal gland　肾上腺

zona glomerulosa　球状带

mineralocorticoid　盐皮质激素

aldosterone　醛固酮

zona fasciculata　束状带

glucocorticoid　糖皮质激素

corticosterone　皮质酮

zona reticularis　网状带

chromaffin cell　嗜铬细胞

adrenaline/epinephrine　肾上腺素

norepinephrine/noradrenaline　去甲肾上腺素

pituitary gland　垂体

basophilic cell　嗜碱性细胞

thyrotroph　促甲状腺激素细胞

thyroid stimulating hormone(TSH)/thyrotropin
　促甲状腺激素

adrenocorticotroph cell(ACTH)/corticotroph
　促肾上腺皮质激素细胞

adrenocorticotropin　促肾上腺皮质激素

gonadotroph　促性腺激素细胞

adenohypophysis　腺垂体

pars distalis　远侧部

acidophilic cell　嗜酸性细胞

somatotroph　生长激素细胞

somatotropin/growth hormone(GH)　生长激素

mammotroph/prolactin cell　促乳激素细胞

mammotropin　促乳激素

follicle stimulating hormone(FSH)　促卵泡激素

luteinizing hormone(LH)　黄体生成素

interstitial cell stimulating hormone(ICSH)　间
　质细胞刺激素

chromophobe cell　嫌色细胞

pars intermedia　中间部

melanotroph　促黑素激素细胞

melanocyte stimulating hormone(MSH)　黑素细
　胞刺激素

pars tuberalis　结节部

neurohypophysis　神经垂体

pars nervosa　神经部

pituicyte　垂体细胞

Herring body　赫林体

hypothalamus　下丘脑

supraoptic nucleus　视上核

paraventricular nucleus　室旁核

vasopressin(VP)　加压素

antidiuretic hormone(ADH)　抗利尿激素

oxytocin(OT)　催产素

infundibulum　漏斗

皮　肤

skin　皮肤

epidermis　表皮

dermis　真皮

hair follicle　毛囊

hair papilla　毛乳头

hair root　毛根

hair shaft　毛干

horny cell　角质细胞

stratum basale　基底层

stratum spinosum　棘层

stratum granulosum　颗粒层

stratum lucidum　透明层

stratum corneum　角质层

melanocyte　黑素细胞

Langerhans cell　朗格汉斯细胞

papillary layer　乳头层

reticular layer　网织层

hypodermis　皮下组织

sweat gland　汗腺

sebaceous gland　皮脂腺

男性生殖系统

male reproductive system　男性生殖系统

testis　睾丸

tunica albuginea　白膜

seminiferous tubule　生精小管

interstitial tissue　间质

spermatogenic epithelium　生精上皮

spermatogenic cell　生精细胞

spermatogonium　精原细胞

primary spermatocyte　初级精母细胞

secondary spermatocyte　次级精母细胞

spermatid　精子细胞

flagellum　鞭毛

spermatozoon　精子

sustentacular cell　支持细胞
testicular interstitial cell　睾丸间质细胞
androgen　雄激素
ductuli efferentes　输出小管
ductus epididymidis　附睾管
epididymis　附睾
prostate gland　前列腺
prostatic concretion　前列腺凝固体

女性生殖系统

female reproductive system　女性生殖系统
ovary　卵巢
superficial epithelium　表面上皮
ovarian cortex　卵巢皮质
ovarian medulla　卵巢髓质
hilus cell　门细胞
follicle　卵泡
primordial follicle　原始卵泡
primary oocyte　初级卵母细胞
oogonium　卵原细胞
follicular cell　卵泡细胞
primary follicle　初级卵泡
zona pellucida　透明带
corona radiata　放射冠
secondary follicle　次级卵泡
follicular cavity　卵泡腔
follicular fluid　卵泡液
cumulus oophorus　卵丘
stratum granulosum　颗粒层
theca folliculi　卵泡膜
theca interna　卵泡膜内层
theca externa　卵泡膜外层
mature follicle　成熟卵泡
secondary oocyte　次级卵母细胞
polar body　极体
first polar body　第一极体
secondary polar body　第二极体
ovum　卵子
ovulation　排卵
corpus luteum　黄体
granulosa lutein cell　颗粒黄体细胞
theca lutein cell　膜黄体细胞
progesterone　黄体酮

estrogen　雌激素
corpus lutein of menstruation　月经黄体
corpus lutein of pregnancy　妊娠黄体
corpus albicans　白体
uterus　子宫
perimetrium　子宫外膜
serosa　浆膜
fibrosa　纤维膜
myometrium　子宫肌膜
endometrium　子宫内膜
uterine gland　子宫腺
spiral artery　螺旋动脉
menstrual cycle　月经周期
proliferative phase　增生期
follicular phase　卵泡期
secretory phase　分泌期
luteal phase　黄体期
menstrual phase　月经期

眼 和 耳

eye　眼
eyeball　眼球
fibrous tunic　纤维膜
vascular tunic　血管膜
retina　视网膜
cornea　角膜
corneal epithelium　角膜上皮
anterior limiting lamina　前界层
corneal stroma　角膜基质
posterior limiting lamina　后界层
corneal endothelium　角膜内皮
layers of retina　视网膜的分层
pigment epithelium layer　色素上皮层
rod and cone layer　视杆视锥层
bipolar cell layer　双极细胞层
ganglion cell layer　节细胞层
pigment epithelial cell　色素上皮细胞
visual cell　视细胞
photoreceptor cell　感光细胞
rod cell　视杆细胞
cone cell　视锥细胞
bipolar cell　双极细胞
ganglion cell　节细胞

ear　耳

cochlea　耳蜗

hair cell　毛细胞

membranous disc　膜盘

organ of Corti　柯蒂器

membranous labyrinth　膜迷路

semicircular canal　半规管

osseous labyrinth　骨迷路

phalangeal cell　指细胞

pillar cell　柱细胞

spiral organ　螺旋器

stereocilium　静纤毛

胚 胎 学 总 论

embryology　胚胎学

fertilization　受精

cleavage　卵裂

implantation　植入

morula　桑葚胚

blastocyst　胚泡

germ disc　胚盘

ectoderm　外胚层

mesoderm　中胚层

endoderm　内胚层

fetal membrane　胎膜

chorion　绒毛膜

amnion　羊膜囊

yolk sac　卵黄囊

allantois　尿囊

umbilical cord　脐带

placenta　胎盘

chorion frondosum　丛密绒毛膜

decidua basalis　底蜕膜

颜 面 发 生

heart prominence　心突

branchial arch　腮弓

branchial groove　腮沟

pharyngeal pouch　咽囊

branchial membrane　腮膜

frontonasal prominence　额鼻突

maxillary prominence　上颌突

mandibular prominence　下颌突

nasal placode　鼻板

nasal pit　鼻窝

median nasal prominence　内侧鼻突

lateral nasal prominence　外侧鼻突

median palatine process　正中腭突

lateral palatine prominence　外侧腭突

dysplasia　发育异常

cleft lip　唇裂

oblique facial cleft　面斜裂

cleft palate　腭裂

duplicate defect　重复性缺损

cervical sinus　颈窦

cervical cyst and cervical fistula　颈部囊肿和颈瘘

消化系统和呼吸系统的发生

foregut　前肠

hindgut　后肠

ultimobranchial body　后鳃体

thyroglossal duct　甲状舌管

midgut loop　中肠袢

cloaca　泄殖腔

urogenital membrane　尿生殖膜

anal membrane　肛膜

proctodeum　原肛

hepatic diverticulum　肝憩室

dorsal pancreatic bud　背胰芽

ventral pancreatic bud　腹胰芽

thyroglossal cyst　甲状舌管囊肿

abnormal rotation of intestinal loop　肠袢转位异常

congenital umbilical hernia　先天性脐疝

umbilical fistula　脐瘘

Meckel diverticulum　麦克尔憩室

stenosis or atresia of digestive tract　消化道狭窄或闭锁

congenital megacolon　先天性巨结肠

Imperforate anus　肛门闭锁

biliary atresia　胆道闭锁

annular pancreas　环状胰

laryngotracheal groove　喉气管沟

laryngotracheal diverticulum　喉气管憩室

lung bud　肺芽

tracheoesophageal fistula　气管食管瘘

agenesis of lung　肺不发育

neonatal hyaline membrane disease　新生儿透明膜病

α-fetal protein，αFP 或 AFP　甲胎蛋白

泌尿和生殖系统的发生

nephrotome　生肾节

nephrogenic cord　生肾索

urogenital fold　尿生殖褶

urogenital ridge　尿生殖嵴

mesonephric ridge　中肾嵴

genital ridge　生殖腺嵴

pronephros　前肾

pronephric tubule　前肾小管

pronephric duct　前肾管

mesonephros　中肾

mesonephric tubule　中肾小管

mesonephric duct　中肾管

Wolffian duct　沃尔夫管

metanephros　后肾

ureteric bud　输尿管芽

metanephrogenic blastema　生后肾原基

urogenital sinus　尿生殖窦

horseshoe kidney　马蹄肾

polycystic kidney　多囊肾

ectopic kidney　异位肾

urachal fistula　脐尿瘘

double ureter　双输尿管

extrophy of bladder　膀胱外翻

renal agenesis　肾缺如

pelvic kidney　骨盆肾

rectovesical fistula　直肠膀胱瘘

sexual differentiation　性分化

sexual undifferentiation　性未分化

primary sex cord　初级性索

primordial germ cell，PGC　原始生殖细胞

indifferent gonad　未分化性腺

cortical cord　皮质索

secondary sex cord　次级性索

gubernaculum　引带

cavity of tunica vaginalis　鞘膜腔

vaginal process of testis　睾丸鞘突

paramesonephric duct　中肾旁管

Müllerian duct　米勒管

sinus tubercle　窦结节

sex-determining region Y，SRY　性别决定区 Y

testis-determining factor，TDF　睾丸决定因子

anti-mullerian hormone　抗中肾旁管激素

vaginal plate　阴道板

hymen　处女膜

genital tubercle　生殖结节

labioscrotal swelling　阴唇阴囊隆起

cryptorchidism　隐睾

congenital inguinal hernia　先天性腹股沟疝

hypospadias　尿道下裂

double uterus　双子宫

vaginal atresia　阴道闭锁

hermaphroditism　两性畸形

true hermaphroditism　真两性畸形

male pseudohermaphroditism　男性假两性畸形

female pseudohermaphroditism　女性假两性畸形

congenital deficiency of androgen receptor　先天性雄激素受体缺乏症

testicular feminization syndrome　睾丸女性化综合征

teratoma　畸胎瘤

心血管系统的发生

haemocytoblast　原始血细胞

primitive cardiovascular system　原始心血管系统

cardiac tube　心管

pricardial coelom　围心腔

cardiogenic plate　生心板

dorsal mesocardium　心背系膜

cardiac jelly　心胶质

myoepicardial mantle　心肌外套层

bulbus cordis　心球

sinus venosus　静脉窦

bulboventricular loop　球室襻

endocardiac cushion　心内膜垫

atrioventricular canal　房室管

septum primum　第一房间隔

foramen primum　第一房间孔

foramen secundum　第二房间孔

septum secundum　第二房间隔

foramen ovale   卵圆孔

valve of foramen ovale   卵圆孔瓣

interventricular foramen   室间孔

membranous part of interventricular septum   室间隔膜部

muscular part of interventricular septum   室间隔肌部

bulbar ridge   球嵴

truncus arteriosus   动脉干

aorticopulmonary septum   主动脉肺动脉隔

atrial septal defect   房间隔缺损

ventricular septal defect   室间隔缺损

transposition of aortic and pulmonary trunks   主动脉和肺动脉错位

stenosis of aorta or pulmonary artery   主动脉或肺动脉狭窄

tetralogy of Fallot   法洛四联症

patent ductus arteriosus   动脉导管未闭